ENDOMETRIOSIS

Christopher Sutton MA FRCOG

Professor of Gynaecological Surgery,
University of Surrey,
The Royal Surrey County Hospital,
Guildford, Surrey

Kevin Jones MSc MRCOG MD

Consultant Obstetrican and Gynaecologist,
The Great Western Hospital,
Swindon, Wiltshire

Published by the RCOG Press at the Royal College of Obstetricians and Gynaecologists, 27 Sussex Place, Regent's Park, London NW1 4RG

www.rcog.org.uk

Registered charity no. 213280

First published 2004

ISBN 1 900364 87 5

RCOG Press Editor: Jane Moody

Design: Tony Crowley

Printed by Latimer Trend & Co. Ltd, Estover Close, Estover Road, Plymouth, Devon PL6 7PL

CONTENTS

INTRODUCTION

Endometriosis is an increasingly common gynaecological disorder, confined to women of a reproductive age and limited to *Homo sapiens* and the higher primates. It would appear that an erect posture, although providing advantages in evolutionary terms for defence, hunting and the acquisition of food, also has a disadvantage: under the influence of gravity, an erect posture allows viable endometrial cells that pass through the fallopian tubes during retrograde menstruation to implant in the deeper areas of the female pelvis.

It is a disease that affects a huge number of women throughout the world, and it has been estimated that between 1% and 15% of women who are examined for pelvic pain and infertility may have endometriosis.[1] This is almost certainly an underestimate; the prevalence of the disease quoted in the medical literature ranges between 6% and 45%.[2–4]

The main problem in trying to estimate the true prevalence of this disease is that the diagnosis can only be made with any accuracy by laparoscopic examination of the pelvis. This specialist procedure is only performed on patients who are referred by their general practitioners (GPs) with dysmenorrhoea, dyspareunia, pelvic pain or infertility. However, a great proportion of women regards many of these symptoms as part of 'a woman's lot in life', and many GPs unfortunately react in a similar way, prescribing increasingly stronger painkillers and multiple courses of antibiotics, in the often mistaken belief that pelvic inflammatory disease is the underlying problem. Thus, the time from the first consultation with typical symptoms to the actual establishment of the diagnosis is of the order of seven years.[5] This has important medico-legal implications, and many GPs are currently facing legal action for this delay in diagnosis, particularly if the patient perceives this to be the cause of her unresolved infertility.

If one accepts the premise that retrograde menstruation is the main cause of this disease, then one would expect endometriosis to become increasingly common with an increased exposure to menstruation. Such increases are inherent in the modern tendency for young women to delay childbearing until their late thirties. In ancient Roman times, a young girl would marry at an age of 14–16 years and normally be expected to become pregnant within a few months of marriage. In the absence of any reliable contraception, she would continue to have pregnancies only delayed by breast-feeding, which usually would create a postpartum amenorrhoeic state. Since the average age of death in those times was 35 years, the number of exposures to retrograde flow of endometrial tissue was minimal compared to the number her modern-day counterpart experiences.

It is for this reason that endometriosis is regarded as a modern-day affliction and is often seen as a disease of the more affluent members of society. In recent years, however, this trend has become less evident. With the worldwide increase in the use of laparoscopy to diagnose the condition, it is becoming obvious that endometriosis is not merely a disease of well-to-do Europeans, but that it poses a significant health problem in the Middle East and countries such as Singapore, India, China, and particularly Japan, which may have the highest incidence in the world.[6]

REFERENCES

1   Barbieri RL. Etiology and epidemiology of endometriosis. *Am J Obstet Gynecol* 1990; 162: 565–7.

2   Balasch J, Creus M, Fabregues F, Carmona F, Ordi J, Martinez-Roman S, Vanrell JA. Visible and non-visible endometriosis at laparoscopy in fertile and infertile women and in patients with chronic pelvic pain: a prospective study. *Hum Reprod* 1996; 11: 387–91.

3   Olive DL, Schwartz LB. Endometriosis. *N Engl J Med* 1993; 328: 1759–69.

4   Vercellini ? *et al.* Epidemiology of endometriosis. In: Brosens I, Donnez J, editors. *The current status of endometriosis.* Carnforth: Parthenon Publishing Group; 1993. p. 111–13.

5   Personnel communication (Endometriosis Society)

6   Miyazawa K. Incidence of endometriosis among Japanese women. Obstet Gynecol 1976; 48: 407–9.

CHAPTER 1

Epidemiology and aetiology

Epidemiology

Endometriosis is one of the most common benign conditions found among gynaecological patients. Various estimates suggest that 6–44% of women of a reproductive age have endometriosis.[1] However, as the accurate diagnosis of this condition depends upon laparoscopic examination, the prevalence of endometriosis in the general population is unknown. The variable appearance of endometriotic lesions at laparoscopy and the ability of gynaecologists to recognise these lesions also affect the reported incidence and prevalence. Furthermore, the prevalence of endometriosis varies depending upon the type of hospital-based population investigated. Table 1.1 shows the prevalence data of specific patient groups. It is most commonly found in patients undergoing invest-igations for infertility and chronic abdominal pain.[2] Prevalence is known to vary according to geography[3] and race, with high levels recorded amongst Japanese women.[4] The incidence of this condition is believed to be higher among first-degree relatives of patients.[5]

Table 1.1 clearly demonstrates a wide vari-ation in the reported prevalence of endo-metriosis, often reflecting investigators' biases at the time the studies were undertaken.[6] There are many potential confounding variables when comparing different national and ethnic groups, including availability of health care, access to contraception, cultural patterns of childbearing and the attitude toward menses. Bias can also occur when patients are selected according to their symptoms at presentation. Thus, prevalence will vary depending upon whether pelvic pain in general, or a specific symptom such as dyspareunia or dysmenorrhoea, is used to select patients. The application of laparoscopy has become much more widespread since the early epidem-iological studies were carried out, influencing diagnostic accuracy and accounting for some of the variation seen in the reported range of prevalence. Finally, the ability to diagnose endomet-riosis varies between gynaecologists, especially in recognising the more subtle or atypical lesions, and this is an important factor for general practitioners to consider when referring patients to hospital.

Because of these problems it is difficult to interpret epidemiological studies and arrive at reliable figures to discuss with patients. However, the epidemiological data do tell us that if a woman has a history of abdominal pain, particularly if this is associated with menstruation or subfertility, it is important to refer her to hospital for laparoscopy because, in a significant proportion of cases, she will have endometriosis.

Aetiology

Endometriosis is defined as the occurrence of endometrial glands and stroma outside the uterine cavity. During

Table 1.1 *Prevalence of endometriosis in specific gynaecological patient groups*

Patient population	Prevalence (%)	Year	Authors
Women with lower abdominal pain	15	1991	Mahmood[2]
	71	1991	Koninckx[7]
Infertile women	21	1991	Mahmood[2]
	20–40	1990	Mahmood[8]
Women with pelvic pain and infertility	84	1991	Koninckx[7]
Cases of unexplained infertility	70–80	1977	Kistner[9]
Women with affected first-degree relatives	7	1980	Simpson[10]
	15	1998	Kennedy[11]
Women with surgically removed ovaries	17	1949	DeSanto[12]
	11	2001	Jones[13]
Women undergoing tubal sterilisation	2	1982	Strathy[14]
	6	1991	Mahmood[2]
Gynaecological laparotomy patients	0.1–50	1984	Houston[15]
Hysterectomy patients	25	1991	Mahmood[2]
Women undergoing diagnostic laparoscopy	0–53	1984	Houston[15]
Estimate in women of reproductive age	6–44	1993	Vercellini[1]
	2–10	1990	Barbieri[16]
Estimate in the general population	1	1993	Shaw[17]
	2–5	1991	Haney[6]

the first half of the twentieth century, two theories were proposed to explain how this condition could arise. Sampson's original theory of retrograde menstruation[18] involves the dissemination of viable uterine endometrium into the peritoneal cavity at the time of menstruation. The endometrial cells attach to the peritoneal surface, proliferate, and invade the underlying tissue. Alternatively, endometriotic tissue may arise from *in situ* metaplasia of peritoneal cells lining the pelvis and ovaries.[19–21] That is, mature cells in the pelvis change in morphology and function from one cell type to another, in response to changes in the pelvic microenvironment. Vascular and lymphatic dissemination of endometriotic cells to distant sites may

then take place. The clinical manifestations of endometriosis occur because the ectopic endometrial tissue responds to ovarian hormones and undergoes cyclical changes. Secretions from the endometriotic cells induce a local inflammatory reaction, fibrous adhesion formation and, in the case of deep ovarian implants, the formation of so-called 'chocolate cysts'. In both theories, endometriosis is regarded as a progressive disease, graduating from minimal to severe stages.

Much more recently, the 'endometriosis disease theory' (EDT)[22] has been proposed. In this model, superficial peritoneal lesions arise because of implantation and are regarded as physiological findings,

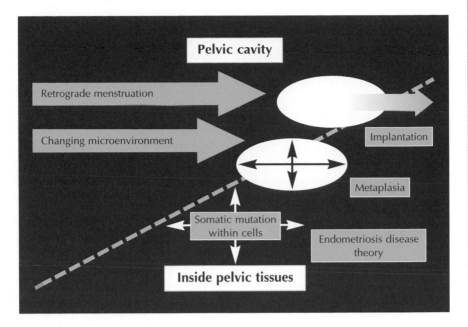

Figure 1.1 *Diagrammatic summary of the theories concerning the origin of endometriotic lesions*

which can regress spontaneously. There is no progression between minimal and severe disease. Severe, deeply infiltrating endometriosis and endometriotic cysts are pathological and arise from somatic mutations within cells, which then develop like a benign tumour. That is, genetic changes occur in predisposed individuals exposed to environmental risk factors such as dioxins and chlorinated biphenyl pollutants. Because these cells are deeply embedded in the pelvic organs they escape the regulatory influence of the peritoneal fluid.

The origin of endometriotic lesions

The theories concerning the origin of endometriotic lesions are summarised in diagrammatic form in Figure 1.1 and include menstrual regurgitation and implantation, the induction theory and the EDT.

Menstrual regurgitation and implantation

In 1927, Sampson first suggested that endometriosis developed following menstrual regurgitation through the Fallopian tubes and subsequent implantation of viable endometrial cells on the surface of the peritoneum.[18] These ectopic cells then proliferate and invade the underlying tissue.[23,24] Sampson's theory is supported by experimental studies,[25] especially by those in which endometriosis develops in the peritoneal cavity of primates following the implantation of menstrual fluid or endometrial tissue.[26,27] However, retrograde menstruation is a common finding in women with normal pelvises; therefore, an additional factor must account for the subsequent development of endometriosis in susceptible individuals. This may be an inability to clear endometrial cells from the pelvis or an inability to prevent them attaching to the peritoneum. A decrease in natural-killer (NK) cell activity leads to a diminished clearance of endometriotic cells, and this immunological mechanism may be important.[28,29] In the Hughesdon hypothesis,[30] endometriotic cysts are thought to originate as a result of the invagination of the ovarian cortex. This is caused by the progressive accumulation of secretions from endometriotic implants on the surface of the ovary, trapped by surrounding adhesions. This concept of an extraovarian pseudocyst has been supported by several studies[31,32] and clinical observations.

Metaplasia of peritoneal cells – the induction theory

Cells lining the Müllerian duct arise from primitive cells, which differentiate into peritoneal cells and the surface cells of the ovaries. In the induction theory, these mature differentiated cells are induced to undergo further metaplastic changes into mature endometrial cells.[19,20] This would also explain the occurrence of endometriosis at any site where Müllerian cells are present. Vascular and lymphatic dissemination of endometriotic cells to distant sites would also occur. The metaplastic change itself may result from stimulation by ovarian hormones or substances secreted by the uterine endometrium, or it may be triggered by an inflammatory irritation (induction concept). Analogous processes have been described for the respiratory epithelium exposed to chronic irritation by cigarette smoke and for the transitional epithelium in the bladder, chronically irritated by calculi, infection or end-metabolites from tobacco smoke excreted in the urine.[21]

Endometriomas may also originate from metaplastic changes of the mesothelium that has invaginated into the ovarian cortex.[33,34] This produces deeply infiltrating ovarian endometriosis and probably accounts for 10% of the 'chocolate cysts', where the ovaries are invariably free. In contrast, endometriomas arising according to the Hughesdon hypothesis are tethered to the posterior surface of the broad ligament by adhesions.

Both the implantation theory and the metaplastic (or induction) theory are widely accepted because they are supported by abundant experimental data.[35]

Endometriosis disease theory

In the implantation and the metaplastic theories, endometriosis is regarded as a progressive disease, developing from minimal to severe stages. In the EDT model, there is no progression from minimal to severe disease.[22] Superficial peritoneal implants are regarded as physiological findings, which can regress spontaneously. However, deeply infiltrating endometriosis and endometriotic cysts are seen as pathological and are believed to arise from cells that have undergone somatic mutations.[36] It is proposed that environmental factors, such as the pollutant, dioxin, cause this somatic mutation in susceptible individuals.[3] The abnormal cells subsequently develop into a benign tumour consisting of endometriotic glands and stroma. Because these cells are deeply embedded in the pelvic organs they escape regulation by the peritoneal fluid.[37] The genetic concept behind EDT is supported by observations of strong familial tendencies.[5,38] and, at a molecular level, by the observation that cystic ovarian endometriosis is clonal in origin.[39]

Factors associated with the development of endometriosis

Genetic factors

There is an increased incidence of endometriosis in first-degree relatives of patients with this disease compared with control groups.[5,11,38] The prevalence of endometriosis can be as high as 15% in the sisters of women with severe disease compared with 1% in the general population. Racial differences also exist, with an increased prevalence reported among Japanese women.[4] It has been suggested that multiple gene loci interact with each other and with environmental factors to predispose an individual to endometriosis.[38]

Environmental factors

Environmental agents, such as dioxin and polychlorinated biphenyl pollutants, have been identified in Belgium as possible cofactors in the development of severe disease.[3] The highest concentrations of these pollutants in breast milk have been found in Belgium, which also has the highest incidence of endometriosis in the world.[3] Much of the endometriosis in this country is of the deeply infiltrating type.

Sociological factors that increase the cumulative menstrual exposure, such as delaying childbearing, also influence the probability of developing endometriosis. For the same reason, drugs such as the combined oral contraceptive pill may be protective.

The peritoneal fluid

The peritoneal fluid is a specific microenvironment containing cytokines, growth factors, prostaglandins and ovarian sex hormones. This fluid is believed to regulate the growth of superficial endometriotic cells.[37] Deep endometriotic lesions, on the other hand, are regulated by blood-stream factors. The depth at which the influence of these two regulators changes over has been estimated to be 5–6 mm.[7]

Immunological factors

Cellular immunity in the endometriotic tissue of women with endometriosis is decreased.[28,29] These women have a lower NK cell activity in both plasma and peritoneal fluid, which correlates with disease severity. However, it is unclear whether this phenomenon is a cause or an effect of endometriosis. Endometrial cells from women with endometriosis also have higher concentrations of P_{450} aromatase, interleukins 6 and 11,[40] heat-shock protein 27,[41] and angiogenesis factors,[42] which are important modulators of cell growth and neo-angiogenesis.

Pathophysiology of pain in endometriosis

It is important to consider, at a pathophysiological level, the mechanisms by which endometriosis can cause pelvic pain. In the early stage of endometriosis, painful symptoms may be caused by the release of mediators, such as prostaglandins, bradykinins, interleukins and the inflammatory products of macrophages, from the endometriotic lesions, altering the receptive properties of the nociceptors in the pelvis.[43,44] In the advanced stages, infiltrating endometriosis results in a direct mechanical compression of the nociceptors, particularly around the uterosacral ligaments.[7,45] In addition, the fibrosis and scarring around the endometriotic implant can induce ischaemic changes resulting in pain. C type pain receptors found in the peritoneum and viscera are activated by chemical and mechanical stimuli. Endometriotic deposits that invade deeply into the underlying tissues may cause mechanical disruption of these fibres leading to pain, or the surrounding local inflammatory response could affect receptor sensitivity.

Pathophysiology of infertility in endometriosis

The pathogenesis of infertility in women with endometriosis is likely to be multifactorial.[46] Women with severe endometriosis have an obvious anatomical distortion of the pelvic organs, for example, periadnexal adhesions or destruction of ovarian tissue by endometriomas. Such distortion may interfere with the release or pick-up of oocytes, and the pain often leads to disorders of coital function. However, the cause–effect relationship between minimal endometriosis and infertility is more difficult to understand, and a large number of possible mechanisms have been suggested.[17,47,48] These include endocrine disorders causing anovulation, such as unruptured luteinised follicle syndrome, prostaglandin-induced luteolysis and oocyte maturation defects. Tubal cilial motility may be altered by prostaglandins from the ectopic endometrium, and uterine endometrial antibodies may interfere with implantation. Endometriosis has also been implicated in male-factor infertility, because it may cause phagocytosis of spermatozoa by activated macrophages. Currently, there is no simple explanation for infertility in the presence of minimal and mild endometriosis.

REFERENCES

1 Vercellini P, Crosignani PG. Epidemiology of endometriosis. In: Brosens IA, Donnez J, editors. *The current status of endometriosis. research and management. Proceedings of the World Congress on Endometriosis, Brussels, June 1992.* Carnforth: CRC Press – Parthenon Publishing Group: 1993.

2 Mahmood TA, Templeton A. Prevalence and genesis of endometriosis. *Hum Reprod* 1991; 6: 544–9.

3 Koninckx PR, Braet P, Kennedy SH, Barlow DH. Dioxin pollution and endometriosis in Belgium. *Hum Reprod* 1994; 9: 1001–2.

4 Miyazawa K. Incidence of endometriosis among Japanese women. *Obstet Gynecol* 1976; 48: 407–9.

5 Kennedy S, Mardon H, Barlow D. Familial endometriosis. *J Assist Reprod Genet* 1995; 12: 32–4.

6 Haney AF. The pathogenesis and aetiology of endometriosis. In: Thomas EJ, Rock J, editors. *Modern approaches to endometriosis.* Lancaster: Kluwer Academic Publishers; 1991. p.113–28.

7 Koninckx PR, Meuleman C, Demeyere S, Lesaffre E, Cornillie FJ. Suggestive evidence that pelvic endometriosis is a progressive disease, whereas deeply infiltrating endometriosis is associated with pelvic pain. *Fertil Steril* 1991; 55: 759–65.

8 Mahmood TA, Templeton A. Pathophysiology of mild endometriosis: review of literature. *Hum Reprod* 1990; 5: 965–70.

9 Kistner RW. Endometriosis. In: Sciarra J, editor. *Gynecology and Obstetrics,* Vol 1. New York: Harper & Row; 1991.

10 Simpson JL, Elias S, Malinak LR, Buttram VC Jr. Heritable aspects of endometriosis. I. Genetic studies. *Am J Obstet Gynecol* 1980; 137: 327–31.

11 Kennedy S, Hadfield R, Westbrook C, Weeks DE, Barlow D, Golding S. Magnetic resonance imaging to assess familial risk in relatives of women with endometriosis. *Lancet* 1998; 352: 1440–1.

12 DeSanto DA, McBirnie JE. Endometriosis – a clinical and pathological study of 219 cases. *Calif Med* 1949; 71: 274–6.

13 Jones JD. The prevalence and age distribution of ovarian cysts among women attending a London teaching hospital. *J Obstet Gynaecol* 2001; 21: 70–1.

14 Strathy JH, Molgaard GA, Coulam CB, Molton LJ 3rd. Endometriosis and infertility: a laparoscopic study of endometriosis among fertile and infertile women. *Fertil Steril* 1982; 38: 667–72.

15 Houston DE. Evidence for the risk of pelvic endometriosis by age, race and socioeconomic status. *Epidemiol Rev* 1984; 6: 161–91.

16 Barbieri RL. Etiology and epidemiology of endometriosis. *Am J Obstet Gynecol* 1990; 162: 565–7.

17 Shaw R. Endometriosis and infertility. In: *Update Postgraduate Centre Series – Infertility.* Oxford: Reed Healthcare Communications; 1995. p.38–43.

18 Sampson JA. Peritoneal endometriosis due to the menstrual dissemination of endometrial tissue into the peritoneal cavity. *Am J Obstet Gynecol* 1927; 14: 422–69.

19 Meyer R. Zur Frage der Urnieren-Genese von Adeno-myomen. *Zentralbl Gynäkol* 1923; 15: 577–87.

20 Meyer R. Über den Stand der Frage der Adeno-myositis und Adenomome im allgemeinen und insbesondere über Adenomyositis seroepithelialis und Adenomyometritis sarcomatosa. *Zentralbl Gynäkol* 1919; 36: 754–63.

21 Fujii S. Secondary Mullerian system and endo-metriosis. *Am J Obstet Gynecol* 1991; 165: 219–25.

22 Koninckx PR, Barlow D, Kennedy S. Implantation versus infiltration: the Sampson versus the endometriotic disease theory. *Gynecol Obstet Invest* 1999; 47(Suppl 1): 3–10.

23 Melega C, Balducci M, Bulletti C, Galassi A, Jasonni VM, Flamigni C. Tissue factors influencing growth and maintenance of endometriosis. *Ann N Y Acad Sci* 1991; 622: 256–65.

24 Olive DL, Schwartz LB. Endometriosis. *N Engl J Med* 1993; 328: 1759–69.

25 TeLinde RW. The background of studies on experimental endometriosis. *Am J Obstet Gynecol* 1978; 130: 570–1.

26 D'Hooghe TM, Bambra CS, Suleman MA, Dunselman GA, Evers HL, Koninckx PR. Development of a model of retrograde menstruation in baboons (Papio anubis). *Fertil Steril* 1994; 62: 635–8.

27 D'Hooghe TM, Bambra CS, Raeymaekers BM, De Jonge I, Lauweryns JM, Koninckx PR. Intrapelvic injection of menstrual endometrium causes endo-metriosis in baboons (Papio cynocephalus and Papio anubis). *Am J Obstet Gynecol* 1995; 173: 125–34.

28 Ishimura T, Masuzaki H. Peritoneal endometriosis: endometrial tissue implantation as its primary etio-logic mechanism. *Am J Obstet Gynecol* 1991; 165: 210–14.

29 Hill JA. Immunology and endometriosis. Fact, artifact, or epiphenomenon? *Obstet Gynecol Clin North Am* 1997; 24: 291–306.

30 Hughesdon PE. The structure of endometrial cysts of the ovary. *J Obstet Gynaecol Brit Emp* 1957; 44: 481–7.

31 Brosens IA, Van Ballaer P, Puttemans P, Deprest J. Reconstruction of the ovary containing large endometriomas by an extraovarian endosurgical technique. *Fertil Steril* 1996; 66: 517–21.

32 Brosens I. Management of ovarian endometriomas and pregnancy? *Fertil Steril* 1999; 71: 1166–7.

33 Donnez J, Nisolle M, Gillerot S, Anaf V, Clerckx-Braun F, Casanas-Roux F. Ovarian endometrial cysts: the role of gonadotropin-releasing hormone agonist and/or drainage. *Fertil Steril* 1994; 62: 63–6.

34 Donnez J, Nisolle M, Gillet N, Smets M, Bassil S, Casanas-Roux F. Large ovarian endometriomas. *Hum Reprod* 1996; 11: 641–6.

35 Van der Linden PJ. Theories on the pathogenesis of endometriosis. *Hum Reprod* 1996; 11(Suppl 3): 53–65.

36 Koninckx PR, Oosterlynck D, D'Hooghe T, Meuleman C. Deeply infiltrating endometriosis is a disease whereas mild endometriosis could be considered a non-disease. *Ann N Y Acad Sci* 1994; 734: 333–41.

37 Koninckx PR, Kennedy SH, Barlow DH. Endometriotic disease: the role of peritoneal fluid. *Hum Reprod Update* 1998; 4: 741–51.

38 Kennedy S. The genetics of endometriosis. *J Reprod Med* 1998; 43(Suppl 3): 263–8.

39 Jiang X, Hitchcock A, Bryan EJ, Watson RH, Englefield P, Thomas EJ, Campbell IG. Microsatellite analysis of endometriosis reveals loss of heterozygosity at candidate ovarian tumor suppressor gene loci. *Cancer Res* 1996; 56: 3534–9.

40 Noble LS, Simpson ER, Johns A, Bulun SE. Aromatase expression in endometriosis. *J Clin Endocrinol Metab* 1996; 81: 174–9.

41 Ota H, Igarashi S, Hatazawa J, Tanaka T. Distribution of heat shock proteins in eutopic and ectopic endometrium in endometriosis and adenomyosis. *Fertil Steril* 1997; 68: 23–8.

42 Hii LL, Rogers PA. Endometrial vascular and glandular expression of integrin alpha(v)beta(3) in women with and without endometriosis. *Hum Reprod* 1998; 13: 1030–5.

43 Vernon MW, Beard JS, Graves K, Wilson EA. Classification of endometriotic implants by morphologic appearance and capacity to synthesise prostaglandin F. *Fertil Steril* 1986; 46: 801–6.

44 Perper MM, Nezhat F, Goldstein H, Nezhat CH, Nezhat C. Dysmenorrhea is related to the number of implants in endometriosis patients. *Fertil Steril* 1995; 63: 500–3.

45 Cornillie FJ, Oosterlynck D, Lauweryns JM, Koninckx PR. Deeply infiltrating pelvic endo-metriosis: histology and clinical significance. *Fertil Steril* 1990; 53: 978–83.

46 Thomas EJ. Endometriosis and infertility. In: Thomas EJ, Rock J, editors. *Modern Approaches to Endo-metriosis*. Lancaster: Kluwer Academic Publishers; 1991. p.113–28.

47 Brosens I. Endometriosis related to infertility. *Curr Opin Obstet Gynecol* 1991; 3: 205–10.

48 Ingamells S, Thomas EJ. Infertility and endometriosis. In: Shaw RW, editor. *Endometriosis – Current Understanding and Management*. Oxford: Blackwell Science; 1995. p.147–67.

7

CHAPTER 2

Diagnosis

Endometriosis is essentially a disease of symptoms, and clinical signs are more difficult to elicit. Advanced cases with a fixed pelvis are an exception. These are usually associated with ovarian endometriomas (also known as 'chocolate cysts') or with nodular deposits in the rectovaginal septum and thickening of the uterosacral ligaments. Unfortunately, the leading symptoms, dysmenorrhoea and pelvic pain unrelated to the menstrual cycle, are extremely common,[1,2] and general practitioners will routinely encounter many young women and girls with these symptoms in their clinical practice. The combination of a relatively common presenting symptom and the absence of any specific blood test or easy method of diagnostic imaging means that

most patients are initially treated with analgesics or a provisional diagnosis of pelvic inflammatory disease is made. Hospital referral is then only considered after repeatedly failing to cure the pelvic pain with multiple courses of medication.

Daniel O'Connor diagnosed endometriosis via laparoscopy in 10% of all new patients seen by him, and one in 20 of the sufferers was a teenager.[3] The symptoms, in order of their occurrence in this patient series from Brisbane, Australia, are shown in Table 2.1. Surprisingly, 155 of 717 patients (22%) had no symptoms at all, while 39 of 717 (5%) had all the significant symptoms of endometriosis – dysmenorrhoea, dyspareunia, pelvic pain and infertility.

Dysmenorrhoea

Dysmenorrhoea is the cardinal symptom of endometriosis and is present in about 85% of women with this condition. Characteristically, there is a congestive phase of pelvic discomfort, which can be present for a few hours before the cramping pain begins, but which is often felt for several days. Indeed, in some women this congestive phase can gradually increase during the second half of the menstrual cycle from the time of ovulation. Some women are able to identify the discomfort that characteristically occurs at the time of ovulation in one or other iliac fossa and then develop a pelvic ache, which gradually increases until menstruation begins.

The severe spasmodic dysmenorrhoea, largely due to prostaglandin release and its resulting uterine contractions, can be relentless and many patients retire to bed with strong analgesics and often place a

Table 2.1 *Symptoms ranked according to their number of occurrences in the Brisbane series.[3] No other symptom of significance occurred in more than one woman*

Symptoms	Women affected (n)
Dysmenorrhoea	227
Dyspareunia	188
No symptoms	155
Infertility	131
Pelvic pain	114
Menorrhagia	105
Altered menstrual cycle	72
Pelvic mass	8
Bowel symptoms	3
Bladder symptoms	2
Galactorrhoea	2

hot-water bottle on the lower abdomen; occasionally, patients actually have permanent disfigurement from repeated scalding, which is a reflection of just how severe the pain can be. Characteristically, the early menstrual cycles following the menarche are anovulatory and, thus, tend to be painless, but we increasingly see young women who have had severe dysmenorrhoea commencing with the very first menstrual cycle. The youngest recorded case of endometriosis occurred in a ten-year-old girl.[4]

It has traditionally been taught that dysmenorrhoea altered as the endometriosis became worse, but data from the Brisbane series[3] show that 101 of the 227 women complaining of dysmenorrhoea had been doing so since the menarche. On closer questioning, many women believed that the quality of the pain had not altered, but the quantity had increased. O'Connor found that when he looked at the adolescents in his series, the striking feature was that the majority (27 out of 35) had suffered from severe dysmenorrhoea since the menarche, and he recommended that a girl who had suffered from severe dysmenorrhoea since her period started, with no abatement, should undergo laparoscopic investigation to exclude endometriosis. Laparoscopy is the 'gold standard' in the diagnosis of endometriosis, and peritoneal implants will not be seen on a computer-assisted tomography (CAT) scan or even by magnetic resonance imaging (MRI).

The actual incidence of dysmenorrhoea is difficult to assess and depends upon many complex and variable factors, including prevailing social and sexual attitudes in different societies. Probably the best population study comes from the Swedish town of Gothenburg, where two GPs, Drs Andersch and Milsom,[5] took a random sample (one in four) of the total female population aged 19 years, residing in Gothenburg. This sample amounted to a total of 2621 women. The doctors received a very large response to their postal questionnaire (90.9%), and they found that 73% of the respondents suffered from primary dysmenorrhoea, while 15% had severe dysmenorrhoea that affected their working ability and could not be controlled adequately by analgesics or ovulation suppression. Regular analgesic consumption was reported by 38.2%, 21.5% used the oral contraceptive pill (initially prescribed for dysmenorrhoea) and a further 17% required analgesia as well as ovulation suppression with the oral contraceptive pill. Twenty-two percent of these women had consulted a GP because of the severity of the dysmenorrhoea and 24% requested further investigation and hospital treatment, because of the failure of symptom relief with analgesics and ovulation suppressants.

It is obvious from the above study that dysmenorrhoea is a common reason for young women and girls to consult their GPs. It is evident from reading the results of the Brisbane series[3] that all women with dysmenorrhoea who do not respond to simple analgesics or antiprostaglandins should undergo laparoscopic examination to exclude endometriosis, especially in the adolescent years when dysmenorrhoea is sufficient to incapacitate them on a monthly basis with respect to school, work, or play. According to O'Connor, "it is rare for idiopathic dysmenorrhoea to cause prolonged progressive incapacity in the absence of serious and obvious psychological problems. No woman should be labelled as psychologically disturbed, however, until laparoscopy at least has been employed to exclude endometriosis".

In 1994, the National Endometriosis Society in the United Kingdom conducted a survey among their members and found that the delay from first presentation to the GP to the final diagnosis by laparoscopy at the referring hospital was on average seven years [personal communication, National Endometriosis Society, UK]. These findings have recently been supported by a study carried out in Brazilian women.[6] It is, therefore, important for the GP to listen carefully to the patient's history, looking out for clues that the pelvic pain or dysmenorrhoea may be due to endometriosis, even at a relatively young age, and not merely to dismiss the patient's menstrual cramps as part of 'a woman's lot'.

Dyspareunia

Of the 717 patients in O'Connor's Brisbane series, 668 women were, or had been, sexually active and, of these women, 188 (28%) admitted to dyspareunia.[3]

Dyspareunia is usually felt during intercourse, particularly in any coital position that facilitates deep penetration. The pain is usually fairly localised and can be quite severe, especially in women with deposits in the rectovaginal septum and uterosacral ligaments, to the point that most women will cry out and suggest a change of position. In some women, the pain is so severe that they avoid intercourse altogether. This can cause considerable psychological problems within a marriage, particularly if the couple is trying for a pregnancy.

The pain changes in nature after intercourse and is often described as a dull ache, which can last for a few minutes to several hours, but it is rare, in our experience, for patients to have pain the following day. This is by no means a hard and fast rule and, certainly, some patients with endometriosis can suffer discomfort the following day, but these patients may have associated venous congestion as part of the pelvic congestion syndrome.[7] Occasionally, these conditions can coexist or be found separately at the time of diagnostic laparoscopy.

Dyschezia and rectal bleeding

Whenever a woman complains of deep dyspareunia one should always enquire about the existence of pain when opening her bowels at the time of menstruation (dyschezia) and also enquire whether there is any rectal bleeding at this time. Examination should include palpation of the rectovaginal septum and the posterior fornix, to ascertain if there is any nodularity in that region. Speculum examination should also be performed to see if there is some evidence of a blue domed cyst in the posterior fornix.

No symptoms

It is interesting to note that one-fifth of the women in the Brisbane series[3] had no symptoms at all, and the disease was diagnosed coincidentally during other surgical procedures, particularly laparoscopic sterilisation. Endometriosis is often referred to as an enigmatic disease, and one of the greatest enigmas is that some women with very small active lesions – scored as 0–5 on the American Fertility Society (AFS) score and placed in the minimal disease category – often complain of excruciating pain, whereas some women found to have stage IV endometriosis with large endometriomas and a completely fixed, solid pelvis, present with infertility problems rather than a complaint of pelvic pain as such.[8]

Pelvic pain

Non-specific pelvic pain, unrelated to the menstrual cycle, occurred in 16% of the patients in the Brisbane series.[3] Although most women with endometriosis will describe congestive pelvic pain starting from a few hours to up to ten days before menstruation and others will describe a pain at the time of menstruation there is a group of women with endometriosis who have pain throughout the cycle. This pain is quite different from the pain of dysmenorrhoea, yet it does interfere with the woman's lifestyle, requiring regular analgesics and, in some cases, even causing incapacity or inability to perform normal daily routines.

It is important to realise that the severity of the pain is not related to the severity of the score on the revised AFS scale.[9] This scale was designed purely to provide an assessment of the likelihood of the disease causing infertility and the clinician must be aware that the attainment of a high numerical grade on a scoring system does not necessarily correlate with the degree of pain experienced by the woman. Studies have shown that the pain in endometriosis is linked to prostaglandin (PG) metabolism, particularly PG-F.[10] Even small lesions are capable of producing large amounts of PG-F and this may account for the finding that women with mild or moderate disease on the AFS scale can often be in more pain than those with extensive disease that may score stage IV on the AFS scale but is largely 'burnt out' and inactive.

Differential diagnosis – other causes of pelvic pain

It is also important to realise that there are other causes of pelvic pain, such as those listed in Table 2.2.

Laparoscopy will usually rule out pelvic inflammatory disease (PID), with intense hyperaemia and pus coming out of the fimbrial ends of the tubes, which should be cultured for *Chlamydia*, anaerobes, and gonococci. Chronic PID will manifest itself as hydrosalpinges, usually with adnexal adhesions. Laparoscopic inspection of the liver and dome of the diaphragm will often reveal the violin-string adhesions of the Fitz-Hugh–Curtis syndrome, which is most often due to a past infection of the pelvis with *Chlamydia trachomatis*,[11] although it was originally described in association with a gonococcal infection.[12] Laparoscopy may not necessarily rule out adenomyosis, and because this is due to islands of endometriotic tissue within the myometrium, the pelvic cavity looks normal at laparoscopy. The diagnosis can occasionally be suggested by a magnetic resonance imaging scan showing changes in the junctional zone, but it is usually made retrospectively by a histological examination of the uterus after hysterectomy. Clinically, this disease can be detected by the presence of a slightly enlarged uterus, which is definitely tender on bimanual examination, particularly during or around the time of the menstrual period. Women with adenomyosis often present with menorrhagia and sometimes

Table 2.2   *Pathological causes of chronic pelvic pain*

Gynaecological cyclical	**Gastrointestinal**
Primary dysmenorrhoea	Irritable bowel syndrome
Secondary dysmenorrhoea	Inflammatory bowel disease
Endometriosis	Constipation
Adenomyosis	Diverticulitis
Pelvic congestion syndrome	Hernia
Ovarian remnant syndrome	Abdominal angina
Chronic functional cyst formation	Recurrent partial obstruction
Asherman syndrome	Malabsorbtion syndromes
Cervical stenosis	Recurrent appendiceal colic
Imperforate hymen	Carcinoma
Uterovaginal anomalies	Referred pain from upper abdominal pathology
Mittelschmerz (mid-cycle)	
	Neurological
Gynaecological non-cyclical	Nerve entrapment syndrome
Adhesions	Neuroma
Chronic pelvic inflammatory disease	Neurofibromatosis
Endometriosis	
Ovarian remnant syndrome	**Musculoskeletal**
Pelvic congestion syndrome	Arthritis and degenerative spine change
Pelvic floor prolapse	Osteoporosis
Neoplasms (for example, leiomyoma or ovarian cysts)	Coccydynia
	Scoliosis/kyphosis and congenital anomalies
	Neoplasms
Genitourinary	
Recurrent urinary tract infections	**Miscellaneous**
Interstitial cystitis	Abdominal migraine
Urethral syndrome	Acute intermittent porphyria
Outflow obstruction	Aneurysm
Pelvic kidney	Herpes zoster
Carcinoma	Sickle cell disease
	Infectious diarrhoea

also with premenstrual spotting. The exact reason for the latter symptom is difficult to explain.[13]

It is important to rule out other causes of pelvic pain, such as the pelvic congestion syndrome.[7] Usually, the intensely engorged veins supplying the ovary and coursing through the back of the broad ligament are very obvious at laparoscopy and can be confirmed by venography. It is also important to rule out other causes of pelvic pain, especially those of the urinary or gastrointestinal tract. Bladder endometriosis sometimes manifests itself by cyclical haematuria and dysuria.

Occasionally, but rarely, the endometriosis infiltrates the area around the ureter causing ureteric obstruction with hydro-ureter, hydronephrosis and loin pain. Cyclical rectal bleeding usually means that the endometriotic lesion has infiltrated through all layers of the rectum or colon and, in rare instances, can be a cause of intestinal obstruction.

Extrapelvic endometriosis has been identified in virtually every organ system and tissue in the body, with the exception of the spleen.[14] It can occur in surgical scars, particularly following a hysterotomy for a mid-trimester termination, but is also seen in the abdominal wound of a caesarean section or hysterectomy. It has even been found in the vaginal vault following vaginal hysterectomy and in an episiotomy scar. Endometriosis is occasionally seen in the umbilicus without prior surgery and presumably implants there by lymphatic spread. It has also been observed in the laparoscopy scar, probably arising at this site by direct implantation of viable endometrial cells carried there when the insufflating gas is released on removal of the primary trochar. The implants present as monthly pain, sometimes with bright red bleeding or a brownish discharge of haemosiderin. Rarely, but dramatically, it can present as cyclical haemoptysis from implants in the lungs or pleura.

Many of the women in our five-year follow-up study[15] who failed to improve after laparoscopic laser surgery were found to have no visible endometriosis at all at the time of a second-look laparoscopy. It transpired that a large proportion of these women had irritable bowel syndrome, the pain of this condition being remarkably similar to that of endometriosis, and there is some evidence that these conditions coexist in a number of women.

Back pain is rarely due to endometriosis, although, if the ovaries are involved with 'chocolate cysts', then the pain is characteristically referred to the region of the upper buttock on the affected side or bilaterally if both ovaries are involved. Sometimes, when the ovary is adherent to the pelvic sidewall by endometriosis, the woman complains of referred pain down the anterior or lateral side of the thigh, but this pain rarely extends below the knee. This pain is due to irritation of the ilio-inguinal nerves as they course around the pelvic sidewall, which is very close to the region just above the ureter where the ovary characteristically becomes adherent.

Infertility

There has been considerable controversy in recent years over the association of the milder forms of endometriosis with infertility. Many researchers have suggested that it is a casual association, which happens to be present at the time of diagnostic laparoscopy performed as part of an infertility assessment, rather than actually a causal relationship. Nevertheless, in the Brisbane series,[3] 131 patients specifically complained of infertility at the time of the initial consultation and the majority of these women were complaining of primary infertility.

There is little doubt that severe endometriosis, with large endometriomas of the ovary and the gross distortion of the tube that is invariably patent but unable to function effectively because it is swollen and stretched over the enlarged ovary, is causally linked to infertility. In these cases, there is usually a considerable amount of endometriotic adhesions, and the dyspareunia caused by endometriosis can be an additional infertility factor. For further information on the relationship of infertility with endometriosis and the efficacy of fertility-enhancing procedures performed by laparoscopic surgery, the reader is referred to Chapter 5.

Clinical signs

Not all women will exhibit clinical signs on examination, and it is noteworthy that 33 of the 717 patients in the Brisbane series, amounting to 5% of the total sample, had

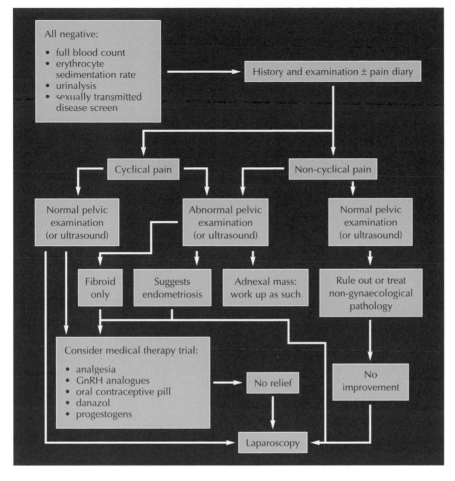

Figure 2.1 *Conventional investigations for endometriosis (with permission)*

neither signs nor symptoms.[3] Nevertheless, most women will be found to be tender when the cervix is gently rocked forward, and this sign of cervical excitation can also be elicited in women with pelvic inflammatory disease. A careful check should be made for any nodularity in the rectovaginal septum, fixity of the pelvic organs and tenderness and nodularity or thickening in the uterosacral ligaments.

Some authorities believe that a pelvic examination is best performed either during

menstruation or just before. In practice, however, depending upon their cultural background, some women may find this slightly distasteful and it often requires tact and a careful explanation as to why this is the time when most information can be obtained. In Belgium, which has the highest incidence of endometriosis in the world, much of it being of the deeply infiltrating type in the uterosacral ligaments and rectovaginal septum, physicians are exceptionally insistent that the examination should be performed at the time of menstruation. It is particularly important if a woman has cyclical rectal bleeding or cyclical haematuria that colonoscopy or cystoscopy is performed during the time of menstruation when the tissue is actively bleeding, otherwise the diagnostic inspection is likely to be negative.

The conventional investigations of chronic pelvic pain are shown in Figure 2.1.

REFERENCES

1 Zondervan KT, Yudkin PL, Vessey MP, Dawes MG, Barlow DH, Kennedy SH. The prevalence of chronic pelvic pain in women in the United Kingdom: a systematic review. *Br J Obstet Gynecol* 1998; 105: 93–9.

2 Zondervan KT, Yudkin PL, Vessey MP, Dawes MG, Barlow DH, Kennedy SH. Prevalence and incidence in primary care of chronic pelvic pain in women: evidence from a national general practice database. *Br J Obstet Gynaecol* 1999; 106: 1149–55.

3 O'Connor DT. Clinical features and diagnosis of endometriosis. In: O'Connor DT, editor. *Endometriosis*. London: Churchill Livingstone; 1987. p.68–84.

4 Houston DA. Evidence for the risk of endometriosis by age, race and socioeconomic status. *Epidemiol Rev* 1984; 6: 167–89.

5 Andersch B, Milsom I. An epidemiologic study of young women with dysmenorrhea. *Am J Obstet Gynecol* 1982; 144: 655–60.

6 Arruda MS, Petta CA, Abrâo MS, Penetti-Pinto CL. Time elapsed from onset of symptoms to diagnosis of endometriosis in a cohort study of brazilian women. *Hum Reprod* 2003; 18: 756–9.

7 Beard RW. Chronic pelvic pain. *Br J Obstet Gynaecol* 1998; 105: 8–10.

8 Vercellini P, Trespidi L, De Giorgi O, Cortesi I, Parazzini F, Crosignani PG Endometriosis and pelvic pain: relation to disease stage and localisation. *Fertil Steril* 1996 65: 299–304

9 American Fertility Society. Revised American Fertility Society classification of endometriosis: 1985. *Fertil Steril* 1985; 43: 351–2.

10 Vernon MW, Beard JS, Graves K, Wilson EA. Classification of endometriotic implants by morphologic appearance and capacity to synthesise prostaglandin F. *Fertil Steril* 1986; 46: 801–6.

11 Wang SP, Eschenbach DA, Holmes KK, Wager G, Grayston JT. Chlamydia trachomatis infection in Fitz–Hugh–Curtis syndrome. *Am J Obstet Gynecol* 1980; 138: 1034–8.

12 MacLean AB. Pelvic Infection. In: Edmonds DK, editor. *Dewhurst's Textbook of Obstetrics and Gynaecology for Postgraduates*, 6th ed. Location: Blackwell; 1999. p.393–409.

13 Wentz AC. Premenstrual spotting: its association with endometriosis but not luteal phase inadequacy. *Fertil Steril* 1980; 33: 605–7.

14 Markham SM, Carpenter SE, Rock JA. Extrapelvic endometriosis. *Obstet Gynecol Clin North Am* 1989; 16: 192–219.

15 Sutton CJG, Hill D. Laser laparoscopy in the treatment of endometriosis. A five-year study. *Br J Obstet Gynaecol* 1990; 97:181–5.

ENDOMETRIOSIS

CHAPTER 3

Investigation

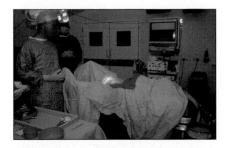

Laparoscopy

Laparoscopy is a surgical procedure in which an optical telescope is inserted into the abdomen in order to view the internal structures (Figure 3.1 a – g). It is currently the 'gold standard' diagnostic test for endometriosis. The operation has been in general use for the visual diagnosis of pelvic pain and infertility for the past 40 years. However, since it is necessary to perform a laparoscopy in order to diagnose endometriosis with certainty, we feel it makes sense to treat the disease at the same time.

In the United Kingdom, laparoscopic laser surgery was first performed at Saint Luke's Hospital in Guildford, in October 1982 by Professor Sutton.[1,2] This is also where the world's first double-blind, prospective study comparing laser surgery with expectant management was carried out.[3] The results of this study clearly showed that laser ablation of endometriosis at laparoscopy is an effective treatment in the majority of women, and that it has considerable advantages over the combination of purely diagnostic laparoscopy and medical therapy. Increasingly, even the most severe cases of endometriosis can now be treated during laparoscopic surgery.[4-8] In view of this, we pursue a 'see-and-treat' management philosophy. It is important that general practitioners refer women who may have endometriosis to

Figure 3.1(a) *During insertion of the laparoscope, the patient remains in a horizontal position*

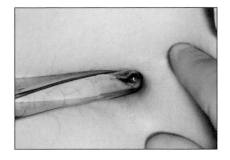

Figure 3.1(b) *An incision is made in the base of the umbilicus*

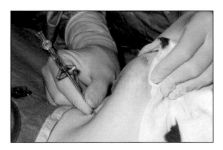

Figure 3.1(c) *The anterior abdominal wall is elevated and the Verres needle inserted*

gynaecologists trained in minimal access surgical techniques. Not only is this cost effective but it will also avoid women having to undergo multiple surgical procedures and should rule out inadequate treatment.

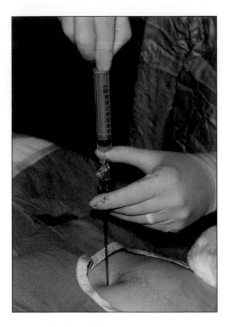

Figure 3.1(d) *A Palmer's test is carried out to confirm the correct placement of the Verres needle*

Technical details of the operation

Laparoscopies are carried out under general anaesthetic and give an excellent view of the pelvic anatomy because they magnify the image (Figures 3.2 and 3.3). The abdominal cavity is inflated with carbon dioxide gas and the laparoscope is introduced through a 5–10 mm long incision inside the umbilicus. Laparoscopy

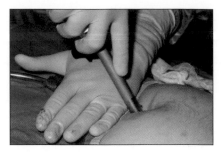

Figure 3.1(e) *The primary tracker is inserted into the distented abdomen*

is generally extremely safe but it is essentially a blind procedure and there is a very small risk, of the order of one in 5000 cases, of damage to the bowel or to one of the major blood vessels. Should this happen, the surgeon would be forced to perform conventional surgery in order to repair any damage.

In addition to the incision in the umbilicus, another 5-mm incision is placed above the pubic hairline in order to insert an irrigator and suction apparatus (Figure 3.4). This allows the surgeon to remove pelvic fluid, to manipulate the pelvic organs in order to examine the pelvis for endometriosis or operate on endometriotic deposits. The CO_2 laser beam is inserted in the right iliac fossa, usually in the line of a bikini mark, as shown in (Figure 3.5 a–d). Some surgeons use bipolar electrical coagulation

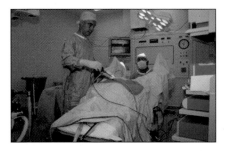

Figure 3.1(f) *Once the laparoscope has been inserted the patient is placed in a 'head down' position*

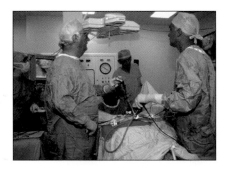

Figure 3.1(g) *The authors performing advanced laparoscopic surgery*

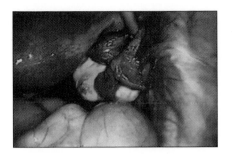

Figure 3.2a *Normal fallopian tube and ovary*

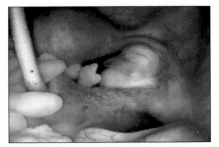

Figure 3.2b *Ovary and fallopian tube floating in saline*

(Figure 3.6) and ultrasonic energy sources (Figure 3.7) to excise or ablate endometriotic deposits. We use the KTP laser to ablate endometriotic cysts (Figure 3.8 a,b). If the procedure is a complicated one, additional 5-mm incisions are made to insert instruments to grasp and hold tissues.

Laparoscopic interventions can vary considerably with regard to operating time. Relatively simple operations may be completed in as little as 20 minutes but the more complicated ones can take two to three hours. If the location of the endometriosis is anticipated to be close to the bowel, it is prudent to ask the woman to take a bowel preparation in order to empty it prior to surgery. This is important because accidental bowel damage would thus be uncontaminated and could be repaired by a surgeon through an open incision.

Postoperative instructions

Some women are treated on a daycare basis or, if the operation is complicated, they may stay in hospital for two to three days. As soon as patients can stamp their feet comfortably, they can undertake all normal activities, including driving a car. They should not, however, engage in strenuous physical activities or heavy lifting for about ten days following the operation, and equally they should refrain from sexual intercourse for the same period of time.

Care of the skin incisions

The small incisions are usually closed with polyglactin 910 (Vicryl®) sutures that dissolve in one to three weeks. Plasters are placed over the wound at the time of the operation and they should be removed after 24 hours. Normal bathing, preferably by a

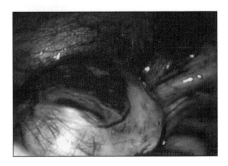

Figure 3.3a *Normal corpus luteum following ovulation*

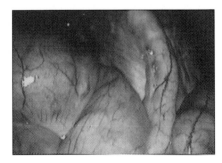

Figure 3.3b *Normal appendix*

19

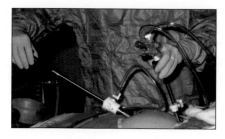

Figure 3.4 *A suction irrigation apparatus is placed suprapubicaly*

shower, is permissible. After this, the wound should be left open, unless it is uncomfortable next to clothing or it is moist, in which case a dry dressing should be placed over it.

Postoperative discomfort and pain

It is quite normal to expect some discomfort after laparoscopic operations. Many

patients report shoulder tip pain due to irritation of the diaphragm by residual carbon dioxide gas or by fluid left in the abdomen to prevent postoperative adhesions. The gas and fluid are normally absorbed within 18–48 hours and the associated pain usually goes away during this time. Patients should get progressively better following laparoscopic surgery, but if they describe increasing abdominal pain and have developed a temperature, the GP should contact the gynaecology team that performed the operation and arrange for readmission of the patient to rule out unsuspected bowel injury.

Urinary problems

Some difficulty may be experienced in passing urine following the operation and

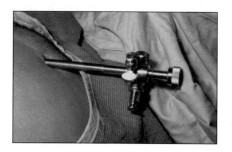

Figure 3.5a *A 7-mm side port for the CO_2 laser is inserted into the right iliac fossa*

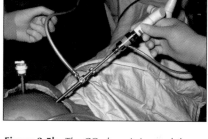

Figure 3.5b *The CO_2 laser is inserted down the port*

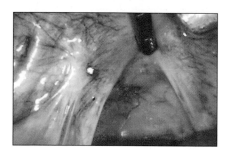

Figure 3.5c *The red spot of the CO_2 laser prior to ablating endometriosis*

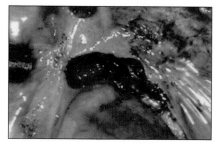

Figure 3.5d *The CO_2 laser ablation of the uterosacral ligaments*

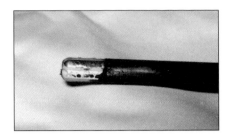

Figure 3.6 *Bicap bipolar diathermy*

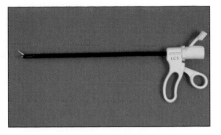

Figure 3.7 *Ultrasonic (harmonic scalpel) shears*

this is because the bladder is usually emptied via a small catheter before the procedure starts. Such discomfort can be managed by drinking an increased amount of fluid, such as barley water or cranberry juice, which alters the acidity of the urine, thus offering some relief. However, if the symptoms persist, then a urinary tract infection should suspected and treated with appropriate antibiotics.

Vaginal bleeding

During the laparoscopy, a small dilator is inserted through the cervix in order to manipulate the uterus. This will result in some postoperative vaginal bleeding, which may last for up to two weeks, and it is not unusual for the woman's periods to be altered during the three months following

any gynaecological procedure. However, if the bleeding is much heavier than a normal period or the discharge becomes offensive, the patients should see their GP, who may prescribe progesterone to suppress bleeding and/or a course of antibiotics.

Laparoscopic appearance of endometriosis

The diagnosis of endometriosis is most commonly made after observing the classical, puckered, black-powder burn lesion with the aid of a laparoscope (Figure 3.9). In addition to these typical lesions, endometriosis has many other laparoscopic appearances, as listed in Table 3.1.[9] Histological examination of these varying types of lesions has identified

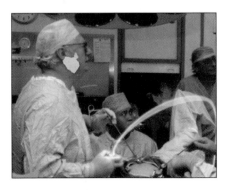

Figure 3.8a *The green light of the KTP laser fibre*

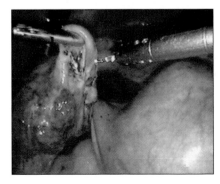

Figure 3.8b *The KTP laser inside the pelvis*

Table 3.1 *The laparoscopic appearance of endometriosis*

- Hyper- or neovascularisation of the peritoneum
- Yellow/brown pigmentation of the peritoneum
- Petechial blood-like red lesions within the peritoneum
- Clear gelatinous lesions (sago grain), usually on the uterus
- Thickened and scarred uterosacral ligaments
- Pseudoperitoneal pockets (Allen–Master's pouch)
- Peritubal adhesions, hydro- or haematosalpinx
- Ovaries adherent to the pelvic side wall and each other
- Obliteration of the pouch of Douglas (often involves bowel adhesions)

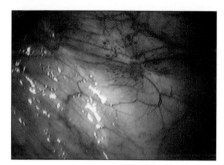

Figure 3.9 *The classical black powder burn lesions indicating endometriotic deposits surrounded by peticheal haemorrhage*

Table 3.2 *Frequency of location of endometriotic implants in the pelvis (from a review of 500 consecutive cases)[9]*

Site	Percentages (%)
Uterosacral ligaments	63.0
Ovaries, superficial	56.0
Ovaries, deep (endometrioma)	19.5
Ovarian fossae	32.5
Anterior vesicle pouch	21.5
Pouch of Douglas	18.5
Broad ligament	7.5
Intestines	5.0
Fallopian tube mesosalpinx	4.5
Salpingitis isthmica nodosa	3.0
Uterus	4.5

endometriotic glands, stroma and fibro-muscular hyperplasia within all such lesions.

The location of endometriosis within the pelvis

Almost all patients have multiple sites within the pelvis that are infiltrated with endometriosis. The most frequent sites of endometriotic involvement, found in a sample of 500 consecutive patients,[9] are summarised in Table 3.2.

There are, however, a number of problems with interpreting this data. We do not know how prevalent endometriosis is in the general female population. The distribution may be quite different in women who are infertile, compared with those who only have pain. Depending on the clinical services offered, different gynaecology units might attract different patient groups. Our unit, for example, offers a tertiary referral service for the surgical treatment of endometriosis, creating a bias towards the most severe forms of the disease, so that pouch of Douglas (Figures 3.10 and 3.11) and recto-

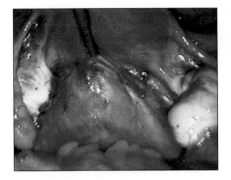

Figure 3.10 *Endometriosis in the pouch of Douglas, tenting the rectum*

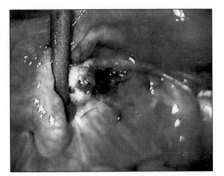

Figure 3.11 *Black deposits of endometriosis behind the ovary*

vaginal septum disease (Figure 3.12a,b) would be relatively more common in a sample of 500 consecutive women examined by laparoscopy in our unit. Operative technique will also affect the apparent distribution of the disease. Endometriosis may be missed at laparoscopy because an inexperienced gynaecologist performs the operation, or because the gynaecologist did not aspirate fluid from the pouch of Douglas and examine the peritoneum covering the ovarian fossa.[10] With advanced endometriosis, the adhesion formation between the reproductive organs and the bowel may make it impossible to identify all the endometriotic lesions. Furthermore, the gynaecologist may fail to take a biopsy to confirm the presence of the disease seen at laparoscopy.

Other investigative techniques

The most severe forms of the endometriosis occur deep within the ovary, the uterosacral ligaments, the rectovaginal septum, in the uterus (adenomyosis) and within the bowel wall. Disease at these sites is not always visible at laparoscopy. Magnetic resonance imaging (MRI), transvaginal sonography (TVS), laparoscopic ultrasound, rectal ultrasound and barium enemas have all been used to detect endometriosis at these sites.

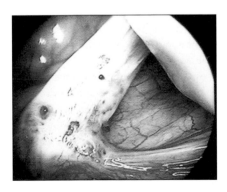

Figure 3.12a *Endometriosis infiltrating the uterosacral ligaments*

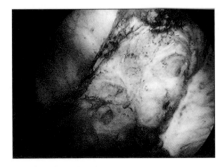

Figure 3.12b *The uterosacral ligaments have been completely ablated by the CO_2 laser*

23

Table 3.3 *Performance of morphological scoring systems in the discrimination between endometriomas and other adnexal masses*

Author	Year	Cysts scanned (*n*)	Sensitivity (%)	Specificity (%)	Positive predictive value	Negative predictive value
Mais[14]	1993	82	84.0	90.0	78.0	93.0
Guerriero[15]	1995	93	83.0	89.0	–	–
Volpi[16]	1995	50	82.4	97.7	94.0	92.8
Dogan[17]	1996	1035	86.5	99.1	91.5	98.2
Alcazar[18]	1997	82	88.9	91.0	84.2	94.5

Magnetic resonance imaging

MRI of the pelvis is a reliable, non-invasive diagnostic test for endometriosis and offers the possibility of screening large numbers of women at risk. It has a sensitivity of 90% and a specificity of 98% for endometriomas[11] and is the only reliable way to diagnose adenomyosis without removing the uterus. It can be difficult to distinguish adenomyosis from intramural fibroids on TVS scans, and MRI scanning has been shown to be significantly better than TVS in the diagnosis of adenomyosis ($P < 0.02$).[12] It is an important distinction to make, because the definitive management of adenomyosis is hysterectomy, whereas fibroids can be treated with the conservation of the uterus.[13] However, MRI is an expensive investigation and it does not form part of the routine investigation of a woman with endometriosis.

Ultrasound

TVS is cheap and readily available. It has been shown to have a high degree of diagnostic accuracy for endometriomas, because it is both sensitive and specific (Table 3.3).

Endometriomas have a characteristic ground-glass appearance on ultrasound, and a preoperative TVS scan should be carried out in all patients suspected of having endometriosis.

TVS has also been used to diagnose adenomyosis preoperativley. The reported sensitivity is 80.0–86.6%, the specificity 50.0–96.2%, the positive predictive value 68.4–86.0% and the negative predictive value 77–98%.[19] The limiting factor in the diagnosis by TVS lies in distinguishing fibroids from adenomyosis.[20] Transrectal ultrasound is being used increasingly and is invaluable in the diagnosis of endometriosis infiltrating the rectal wall and the uterosacral ligaments.[21,22]

Barium enemas

Barium enemas, with and without air contrast vaginograms, can be used to detect endometriotic lesions infiltrating the full thickness of the bowel wall and causing a stricture. When a woman complains of dyschezia or cyclical rectal bleeding, it is important to request this investigation, because she may need an anterior bowel resection at laparotomy or a laparoscopically assisted segmental bowel resection.

Serum markers

The CA125 epitope can be used as a serum marker for endometriosis (detected by the monoclonal antibody, OC-125).[23] This is elevated in women with revised AFS stages III and IV, where the sensitivity and specificity, respectively, are over 80% and 90% if a cut-off level of 35 u/ml is used. However, women with mild and minimal stages of endometriosis have CA125 levels that lie within the normal range. The specificity of serum CA125 as a screen for the presence of endometriosis is consequently poor and it is not in routine clinical use.

Histological diagnosis

Endometriosis is defined by the presence of endometrial glands and stroma outside the uterine cavity. The laparoscopic diagnosis of endometriosis depends on the recognition of the wide range of visual appearances of this disease. Other peritoneal lesions share morphological features similar to those of endometriosis, and the diagnosis is often difficult, especially in women who have had previous surgery. Furthermore, the histopathology of endometriotic tissue varies according to the type of lesion. In one study, endometriosis was histologically confirmed in 57% of the obtained biopsies, while all or some of the biopsies confirmed the diagnosis of endometriosis in 73% of the patients.[24] Superficial peritoneal endometriosis is recognised by the presence of endometrial glands and stroma. However, deep endometriosis is a proliferative lesion composed of fibromuscular tissue with sparse, finger-like extensions of glandular and stromal tissue.[25] The endometrial component varies considerably. This makes histological confirmation problematic. Even when there is no visible evidence of endometriosis at laparoscopy, microscopic deposits can be observed histologically.[26–28] In practice, some surgeons rely on the pathognomonic appearance of the lesion, especially endometriomas, and selectively biopsy tissue when they are suspicious, whilst others routinely take tissue for histological examination. Therefore, neither visual inspection, nor the histological examination of excised tissue will conclusively diagnose endometriosis.

Classification

Because there is no direct correlation between the volume of endometriotic tissue and the severity of symptoms with regard to either pain or infertility, classifying and staging endometriosis is problematic. The different appearances of endometriosis at laparoscopic inspection and the different histological appearances of the lesions also make staging the disease difficult.

A number of classification systems for endometriosis have been described. All these classifications divide endometriosis into various stages, from minimal to severe disease. In an attempt to correlate increasing disease severity with subsequent fertility outcome, the disease score increases with the involvement of the ovaries and with adhesion formation. The revised American Fertility Society (AFS) score[29] is used most commonly in investigative studies and it has the benefit of allowing a comparison between the results reported by different groups (Figure 3.13). However, the majority of women present with pelvic pain as the predominant symptom. Deep retroperitoneal endometriosis is responsible for pelvic pain,[30] and the intensity of the

The American Fertility Society Revised Classification of endometriosis

Patient's Name _____ Date _____

Stage I   (Minimal)   1 – 5
Stage II   (Mild)   6 – 15
Stage III (Moderate) 16 – 40
Stage IV   (Severe)   > 40
Total _____

Laparoscopy _____ Laparotomy _____ Photography _____
Recommended Treatment _____
_____
_____

Prognosis _____

PERITONEUM	**ENDOMETRIOSIS**		< 1 cm	1 – 3 cm	> 3 cm
		Superficial	1	2	4
		Deep	2	4	6
OVARY	R	Superficial	1	2	4
		Deep	4	16	20
	L	Superficial	1	2	4
		Deep	4	16	20

	POSTERIOR CUL-DE-SAC OBLITERATION		Partial		Complete
			4		40

	ADHESIONS		< 1/3 Enclosure	1/3 – 2/3 Enclosure	> 2/3 Enclosure
OVARY	R	Filmy	1	2	4
		Dense	4	8	16
	L	Filmy	1	2	4
		Dense	4	8	16
TUBE	R	Filmy	1	2	4
		Dense	4*	8*	16
	L	Filmy	1	2	4
		Dense	4*	8*	16

* If the fimbriated end of the Fallopian tube is completely enclosed, change the point assignment to 16

Additional Endometriosis: _____

Associated Pathology _____

To be used with normal tubes and ovaries

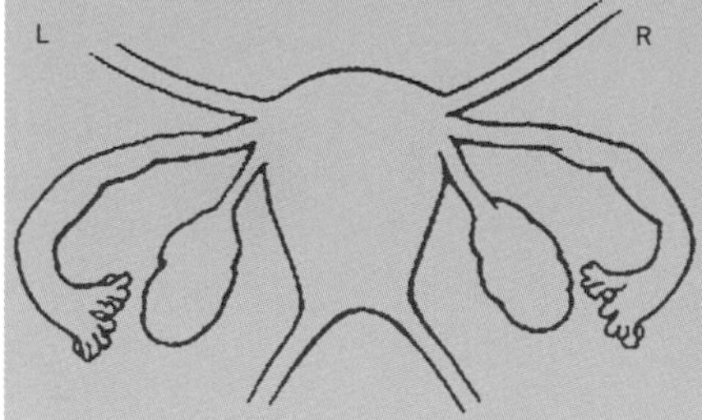

To be used with abnormal tubes and/or ovaries

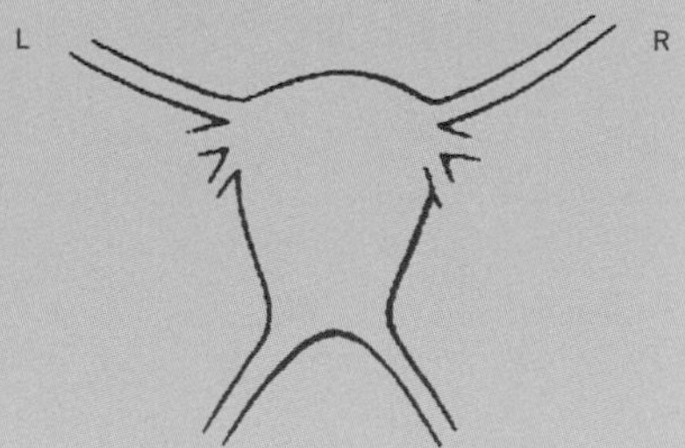

Figure 3.13 *The revised American Fertility Society score (with permission)*

pain is related to the depth to which the lesion penetrates.[31] Therefore, the disease and its treatment need to be assessed in terms of pain, rather than merely in terms of predicting fertility.

The revised AFS recording system gives a high score in the presence of adhesions that may be relevant to infertility, but it does not correlate well with chronic pain.

For example, chronic pain may be due to rectovaginal nodules, which have a low revised AFS score.

REFERENCES

1 Sutton CJG. Initial experience with carbon dioxide laser laparoscopy. *Laser Med Sci* 1985; 1: 25–31.

2 Sutton CJG, Hill D. Laser laparoscopy in the treatment of endometriosis: a five-year study. *Br J Obstet Gynaecol* 1990; 97: 901–5.

3 Sutton CJ, Ewen SP, Whitelaw N, Haines P. Prospective, randomised, double-blind, controlled trial of laser laparoscopy in the treatment of pelvic pain associated with minimal, mild, and moderate endometriosis. *Fertil Steril* 1994; 62: 696–700.

4 Jones KD, Sutton CJG. Laparoscopic management of ovarian endometriomas: a critical review of current practice. *Curr Opin Obstet Gynecol* 2000; 12: 309–15.

5 Daniell JF, Lalonde CJ. Advanced laparoscopic procedures for pelvic pain and dysmenorrhoea. In: Sutton C, *editor. Advanced Laparoscopic Surgery.* London: Balliere–Tindall; 1995. p.795–808.

6 Nezhat C, Nezhat F, Pennington F. Laparoscopic treatment of infiltrative rectosigmoid colon and rectovaginal septum endometriosis by the technique of videolaparoscopy and the CO_2 laser. *Br J Obstet Gynaecol* 1992; 99: 664–7.

7 Donnez J, Nisolle M, Casanas-Roux F, Bassil S, Anaf V. Rectovaginal septum endometriosis or adenomyosis: laparoscopic management in a series of 231 patients. *Hum Reprod* 1995; 10: 630–5.

8 Biggerstaff ED. Laparoscopic surgery for pelvic pain. In: Sutton CJG, Diamond MD, *editors. Endoscopic Surgery for Gynaecologists* (2nd edition). London: WB Saunders; 1998. p.261–71.

9 Shaw R. *An Atlas of Endometriosis.* Leicester: Parthenon Publishing Group Ltd; 1993. p.23–27.

10 Koninckx PR. Biases in the endometriosis literature illustrated by 20 years of endometriosis research in Leuven. *Eur J Obstet Gynecol Reprod Biol* 1998; 81: 259–71.

11 Togashi K, Nishimura K, Kimura I, Tsuda Y, Yamashita K, Shibata T, *et al.* Endometriotic cysts: diagnosis with MR imaging. *Radiology* 1991; 180: 73–8.

12 Ascer SM, Arnold LL, Patt RH, Schruefer JJ, Bagley AS, Semelka RC, *et al.* Adenomyosis: prospective comparison of MR imaging and transvaginal sonography. *Radiology* 1994; 190: 803–6.

13 Goodwin SC, Walker WJ. Uterine artery embolisation for the treatment of uterine fibroids. *Curr Opin Obstet Gynaecol* 1998; 10: 315–20.

14 Mais V, Guerriero S, Ajossa S, Angiolucci M, Paoletti AM, Melis GB. The efficiency of transvaginal ultrasonography in the diagnosis of endometrioma. *Fertil Steril* 1993; 60: 776–80.

15 Guerriero S, Mais V, Ajossa S, Paoletti AM, Angiolucci M, Labate F, Melis GB. The role of endovaginal ultrasound in differentiating endometriomas from other ovarian cysts. *Clin Exp Obstet Gynecol* 1995; 22: 20–2.

16 Volpi E, De Grandis T, Zuccaro G, La Vista A, Sismondi P. Role of transvaginal sonography in the detection of endometriomata. *J Clin Ultrasound* 1995; 23: 163–7.

17 Dogan MM, Ugur M, Soysal SK, Soysal ME, Ekici E, Gokmen O. Transvaginal sonographic diagnosis of ovarian endometrioma. *Int J Gynecol Obstet* 1996; 52: 145–9.

18 Alcazar JL, Laparte C, Jurado M, Lopez-Garcia G. The role of transvaginal ultrasonography combined with colour velocity imaging and pulsed Doppler in the diagnosis of endometrioma. *Fertil Steril* 1997; 67: 487–91.

19 Fedele L, Bianchi S, Dorta M, Arcaini L, Zanotti F, Carinelli S. Transvaginal ultrasonography in the diagnosis of diffuse adenomyosis. *Fertil Steril* 1992; 58: 94–7.

20 Brosens JJ, de Souza NM, Barker FG, Paraschos T, Winston RM. Endovaginal ultrasonography in the diagnosis of adenomyosis uteri: identifying the predictive characteristics. *Br J Obstet Gynaecol* 1995; 102: 471–4.

21 Chapron C, Dumontier I, Dousset B, Fritel X, Tardif D, Roseau G, *et al.* Results and role of rectal endoscopic ultrasonography for patients with deep pelvic endometriosis. *Hum Reprod* 1998; 13: 2266–70.

22 Ohba T, Mizutani H, Maeda T, Matsuura K, Okamura H. Evaluation of endometriosis in uterosacral ligaments by transrectal ultrasonography. *Hum Reprod* 1996; 11: 2014–17.

23 Barbieri RL, Blast RC, Niloff JM, *et al.* Elevation of a serological test for the diagnosis of endometriosis using a monoclonal antibody OC-125. Presented at the Annual Meeting of the Society of Gynecological Investigation, 1985.

24 Shafik A, Ratcliffe N, Wright J. The importance of histological diagnosis in patients with chronic pelvic pain and laparoscopic evidence of endometriosis. *Gynecol Endosc* 2000; 5: 301–4.

25 Brosens I, Vasquez G, Deprest J, Puttemans P. Pathogenesis of endometriosis. In: Nezhat CR, *et al., editors. Endometriosis. Advanced Management and Surgical Techniques.* New York: Springer Verlag; 1995.

26 Nisolle M, Paindaveine B, Bourdon A, Berliere M, Casanas-Roux F, Donnez J. Histologic study of peritoneal endometriosis in infertile women. *Fertil Steril* 1990; 53: 984–8.

27 Redwine DB, Yocum LB. A serial section study of visually normal pelvic peritoneum in patients with endometriosis. *Fertil Steril* 1990; 54: 648–51.

28 Nezhat F, Allen CJ, Nezhat C, Martin DC. Nonvisualised endometriosis at laparoscopy. *Int J Fertil* 1991; 36: 340–3.

29 The American Fertility Society. Revised American Fertility Society classification of endometriosis: 1985. *Fertil Steril* 1985; 43: 351–2.

30 Cornille FJ, Oosterlynck D, Lauweryns JM, Koninckx PR. Deeply infiltrating pelvic endometriosis: histology and clinical significance. *Fertil Steril* 1990; 53: 978–83.

31 Koninckx PR, Meuleman C, Demeyere S, Lesaffre E, Cornillie FJ. Suggestive evidence that pelvic endometriosis is a progressive disease, whereas deeply infiltrating endometriosis is associated with pelvic pain. *Fertil Steril* 1991; 55: 759–65

CHAPTER 4

Medical treatment

Endometriosis is known to regress in pregnancy, under the influence of androgens, and after the menopause. Medical management aims to mimic these states, and the rationale behind the treatment strategies is to induce atrophy of the ectopic endometrium in order to relieve painful symptoms and restore fertility.

Because endometriosis is an oestrogen-dependent condition, drugs that suppress ovarian oestrogen activity, either directly or indirectly by suppressing pituitary function, are widely used. These include danazol, gestrinone and gonadotrophin-releasing hormone (GnRH) analogues. Visible disease and painful symptoms generally regress during physiological amenorrhoeic states, such as the menopause or pregnancy, and drugs that can induce amenorrhoea, such as combined oral contraceptives and the progestogens, are also used in the treatment of endometriosis. The symptomatic relief of pain can be achieved using simple analgesics, such as paracetamol and aspirin, or compound analgesic preparations containing these drugs in combination with low-dose opioid analgesics. The nonsteroidal anti-inflammatory drugs (NSAIDs) are particularly useful in treating dysmenorrhoea. However, a critical review of the medical management of endo-metriosis has shown that there is little difference in the effectiveness of the various treatments, and their use is limited by unacceptable non-therapeutic effects.[1] Furthermore, many of the drugs have a contraceptive action,[2] and this is clearly a disadvantage to a woman who is trying to conceive.

The randomised controlled trials on the surgical treatment of endometriosis have shown that surgery is effective in the management of both painful symptoms and subfertility. Therefore, we recommend that medical treatments are used by general practitioners for the short- to medium-term control of painful symptoms, prior to referral of the woman to hospital or while she is on the waiting list for surgery. Medical therapy alone has no role to play in the management of endometriotic cysts or infiltrating rectovaginal disease, which require surgery.

Drug treatments

Danazol

Danazol was the first pharmaceutical agent used to treat endometriosis and until the advent of gonadotrophin-releasing agents it was also the most commonly used drug. Danazol is a synthetic steroid derived from ethisterone, which inhibits the secretion of pituitary gonadotrophins, thereby suppressing ovarian oestrogen production. It also has direct androgenic, anti-oestrogenic, and antiprogestogenic activity on the endometrium, which usually results in amenorrhoea.[3] Thus, it leads to atrophy of the ectopic endometrium and decreases menstrual loss. The recommended starting dose for treating endometriosis is 200–800 mg daily by mouth, in up to four divided doses, usually for six months. The use of danazol is limited by its androgenic effects, including menstrual irregularity, weight gain, hirsutism, acne, mood changes, changes in libido and, rarely, cliteromegaly and thickening of the vocal chords leading to irreversible hoarseness (for this reason it should not be prescribed to professional singers). It is also contraindicated in women with thromboembolic disease, and it may cause rare hepatic tumours.

Gestrinone

Gestrinone is a synthetic steroid derived from 19-norethisterone. Its mode of action and adverse-effect profile are similar to those of danazol,[4] but it has a longer half-life and only needs to be taken twice weekly. The recommended starting dose for treating endometriosis is 2.5mg by mouth twice weekly, starting on the first day of the cycle with a second dose taken three days later. This should be repeated on the same two days each week, usually for six months.

Gonadotrophin-releasing hormone analogues

There are a number of GnRH analogues used in the treatment of endometriosis, and these are listed in Table 4.1. These drugs are competitive inhibitors of the GnRH receptors in the pituitary gland.[5] After an initial 'flare-up' phase, during which these drugs stimulate pituitary secretion, the production of pituitary gonadotrophins (follicle-stimulating hormone and luteinising hormone) is inhibited or downregulated. Because of this initial stimulation, women should be warned that symptoms might get worse over the first two weeks, before gradually improving. The drugs lead to suppression of ovarian function and anovulation, which reduces circulating oestrogen levels.

This eventually leads to amenorrhoea and to atrophy of the ectopic endometrium. The initial stimulation phase can cause the development of ovarian cysts and menstrual irregularities that may require the treatment to be stopped. In order to avoid this, GnRH analogues are usually commenced during the early part of the menstrual cycle, and the recommended doses are shown in Table 4.1. Unwanted effects of GnRH analogues are related to the low oestrogen levels and include menopause-like symptoms, such as hot flushes, increased sweating, vaginal dryness, dyspareunia and loss of libido. They can also cause local reactions at the site of administration. In the long term, loss of trabecular bone limits the duration of this treatment for endometriosis to six months and it should not be repeated. However, GnRH analogues are increasingly being used for longer periods of time in conjunction with so-called 'add-back hormone replacement therapy'. Bone mineral density in the spine typically

Table 4.1 GnRH analogues used in the treatment of endometriosis. (dosages as recommended in British National Formulary)

Drug	Route of administration	Dosage
Buserelin	Intranasal	300 µg, 3 x day
Nafarelin	Intranasal	200 µg, 2 x day
Triptorelin	Intramuscular	3.0 mg, 1 x month
Goserelin	Subcutaneous	3.6 mg, 1 x month
Leuprorelin	Intramuscular or subcutaneous	3.75 mg, 1 x month

falls by 4–6% with six months of GnRH analogue treatment.[6] Adding a progestogen or an oestrogen reduces the loss of bone mineral density by up to 50%.[7–9] The same effect can be achieved with tibolone (2.5mg daily for six months).[10–12] Use of add-back oestrogen also reduces the incidence of unpleasant menopausal symptoms that occur with GnRH analogue therapy, but it does not affect pain relief.[7,13]

The combination of GnRH analogues with add-back therapy has enabled the physician to produce an amenorrhoeic, pain-free state for long periods of time with minimal adverse effects. The main limiting factor is the expense of the GnRH analogues and the need to arrange follow-up visits for intramuscular or sub-cutaneous injections as well as bone scans. This management strategy also allows the gynaecologist to assess whether or not a patient will benefit from radical surgery with oestrogen therapy postoperatively because the drug regimen effectively produces a 'chemical' hysterectomy and bilateral salpingo-oophorectomy. If the woman is comfortable with this drug regimen, she is likely to benefit from the operation.

Progestogens

There is a range of progestogens[2] that can be used in different ways to treat endometriosis by suppressing endometrial growth (Figure 4.1). The aim is to increase the dose to an amenorrhoea-inducing level, which may also produce atrophy in the ectopic endometrial tissue. Unwanted effects include irregular bleeding, bloating, and weight gain. Medroxyprogesterone acetate and dydrogesterone are the least androgenic of the progestogens. The recommended dose for mild to moderate endometriosis with medroxyprogesterone acetate is 10mg by mouth three times daily for 90 consecutive days, beginning on the first day of the cycle. For dydrogesterone, the manufacturer recommends that oral doses of 10 mg twice or three times daily

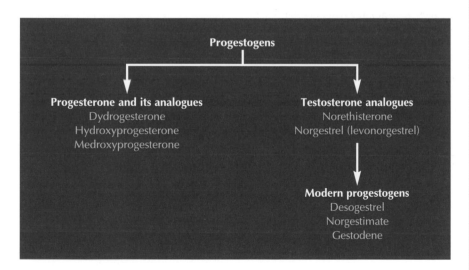

Figure 4.1 *The progestogens*

are used, either on days 5–25 of the menstrual cycle or continuously. Norethistrone has an adverse-effect profile similar to the progesterone analogues but is more virilising. The recommended dose for norethisterone is 10–15mg daily, and this can be increased to 20–25mg/day to suppress spotting if it occurs. The drug is taken by mouth for four to six months or longer, starting on day five of the menstrual cycle.[14]

Contraceptives

Using contraceptives to avoid menstrual bleeding is another strategy often used to control the painful symptoms of endometriosis. The combined oral contraceptive pill (usually ethinyloestradiol at 20–35µg/day plus a progestogen) can be taken continuously (tricycling the combined oral contraceptive) for long periods of time to avoid menstruation. The intrauterine progestogen-only system is a contraceptive device, which is having an increasing impact on the management of dysfunctional uterine bleeding. It consists of a T-shaped intrauterine device sheathed with a reservoir of levonorgestrel that is released at the rate of 20µg per 24 hours (Mirena® system). This prevents endometrial proliferation and thereby reduces both the duration of bleeding and the amount of menstrual loss. The Mirena system has been shown to alleviate painful symptoms and reduce the size of rectovaginal deposits of endometriosis in a prospective clinical trail.[15] It is our experience that it is useful for relieving the symptoms of endometriosis that deeply infiltrates the uterine musculature, so-called adenomyosis. The long-acting, parenteral, progestogen-only contraceptives, medroxyprogesterone acetate and norethistrone enantate, may be useful as well. They may cause menstrual irregularities initially but, if they induce amenorrhoea, this can provide symptomatic pain relief.

It is important to note that non-hormonal, barrier-type methods of contraception should be used whenever danazol, gestrinone, a progestogen, or a GnRH analogue is being taken to treat endometriosis.

Analgesics

Many women do not wish to use hormonal preparations because they are trying to conceive or the adverse affects of treatment are too difficult to cope with. For these women, the symptomatic relief of pain can be achieved using simple analgesics such as paracetamol and aspirin, or compound analgesic preparations containing these drugs in combination with a low-dose opioid analgesic. The NSAIDs are particularly useful for treating dysmenorrhoea. Other strategies might include the use tranexamic acid in combination with NSAIDs to decrease menstrual loss and relieve dysmenorrhoea to a greater extent.

Antispasmodics

Antispasmodic drugs can be tried in women who, at laparoscopy, are judged to have minimal disease and who may have an element of irritable bowel syndrome. However, these drugs have no role to play in the routine management of endometriosis.

Aromatase inhibitors

Aromatase inhibitors are a group of drugs which have been used to treat breast cancer, and they may have a role in the management of endometriosis. The enzyme aromatase is not normally expressed in the endometrium, however it is found in endometriotic stromal cells. The enzyme catalyses the conversion of C19 steroids to oestrogens, which then stimulates cyclooxygenase-2 to incise the levels of PGE_2. PGE_2 in turn is a potent inducer of aromatase activity. The net effect is to establish a positive feedback cycle which increases the levels of the mediators of inflammation and pain.[14,15] Large clinical trials have not been carried out to establish whether this class of drugs has a significant role in medical management of endometriosis .

Medical trials

The clinical evidence for the use of drug therapy is based on trials comparing a particular drug with placebo, or with another drug.[1]

Painful symptoms

There are only four placebo controlled trials reported in the literature which examine the relief of pain. The trials lasted between three and six months and involved 285 women with various stages of endometriosis. One trial assessed medroxy-progesterone acetate (100mg/day) or danazol (600mg/day),[16] two trials assessed the GnRH analogue leuprorelin (3.75mg every four weeks as a depot intramuscular injection),[17,18] and the fourth trial assessed cyclical dydrogesterone (40mg- or 60mg-dose only).[19] Compared with placebo, danazol, medroxyprogesterone acetate, leuprorelin and cyclical dydrogesterone (60mg dose only) provided pain relief while women remained on treatment.

Only one trial demonstrated a lower prevalence of pain relief at 12 months compared to the placebo group.[16]

Comparisons between drugs has also been carried out. A systematic review has collated 15 randomised controlled trials involving 1299 women with endometriosis.[7] In this review Danazol was compared to the GnRH analogues. Various doses of drugs were used and treatment lasted up to six months. There were no differences with respect to pain relief which was relieved equally by both medications, however, Danazol produced more androgenic effects, while GnRH analogues produced menopausal symptoms.

A systematic review[20] has identified one randomised trial of the combined oral contraceptive (ethinyloestradiol 20 micrograms plus desogestrel 150 micrograms) compared with a GnRH analogue (goserelin, 3.6mg every four weeks).[21] The trial involved 57 patients with endometriosis, treatments lasted for six months, and relief of painful symptoms was the main outcome measure. As expected the patients on GnRH analogues became amenorrhoeic, and experienced menopausal symptoms. Both groups of patients experienced significant symptom relief while they took the drugs.

Six months of gestrinone (5.0–7.5mg/weekly) was compared with danazol (600–800mg)[22] in a randomised trial involving 39 women, and to GnRH analogues in a randomised trial involving 55 women.[23] All the medical treatments significantly reduced painful symptoms while the women used the drugs but they were associated with similar rates of recurrence of symptoms during the follow up period.

Fertility

Six months of drug therapy using danazol (400–800mg), buserelin (1.2mg/day), medroxyprogesterone (600mg/day) acetate or gestrinone (5mg/week) in women with subfertility and laparoscopically proven endometriosis did not improve pregnancy rates compared to either placebo or no treatment.[24] In comparisons of danazol with another drugs that suppresses ovarian function, there was no difference between any of the treatments in terms of pregnancy rates.

Endometriotic cysts and severe endometriosis

Only four trials have demonstrated the effect of medical therapy on endometriotic cysts without surgical treatment also being involved. Three trials compared danazol (600–800mg/day) with GnRHa (triptorelin 3.75mg depot every four weeks, or buserelin 1.2mg day intranasally or 200 micrograms subcutaneously). The trials reported a similar reduction in cyst diameter of 40%, 51% and 57%, with no difference between danazol and GnRHa after six months of treatment.[25–27] Another trial demonstrated that a 25% decrease in endometriomal diameter occurred using a GnRHa when compared with placebo.[28] The efficacy of medical therapy alone in relieving painful symptoms, or its effect on pregnancy and cyst recurrence rates in large groups of women has not been reported. Prospective trials have been reported where medical therapy has been used for six months in conjunction with laparoscopic surgery for endometriotic cysts or severe (stage III–IV) endometriosis.[16,29,30] Danazol (600mg/day) or medroxyprogesterone acetate (100mg/day) reduced pain while the women took the medication.[16] Postoperative GnRH analogues (nafarelin 400 micrograms/day) also reduce postoperative pain but the additional benefits of medication do not seem to persist after drug therapy ended.[29,30]

Conclusions

A critical appraisal of these trials has shown that there is little difference in the effectiveness of various medical treatments with regard to pain relief, which only lasted while women remained on treatment. It has also shown that drug therapy does not improve fertility or eradicate endometriotic cysts. The only major differences between the various available drugs lie in the adverse-effect profiles. Therefore, we recommend that medical treatment be prescribed by GPs for the short- to medium-term control of painful symptoms, prior to referral of the woman to hospital for surgery or assisted conception. The choice of medical treatment depends upon several factors in a woman's history, the most important of which are her experience with previous treatments, her age, her fertility plans and the nature and severity of the symptoms she is experiencing.

REFERENCES

1 Farquhar C, Sutton CJG. The evidence for the management of endometriosis. *Curr Opin Obstet Gynecol* 1998; 10: 321–32.

2 Anonymous. Managing endometriosis. *Drug Therap Bull* 1999; 37: 25–9.

3 Anonymous. Danazol – good mainly for endometriosis. *Drug Therap Bull* 1990; 28: 22–4.

4 Anonymous. Gestrinone (dimetriose) – another option in endometriosis. *Drug Therap Bull* 1991; 29: 45.

5 Anonymous. Gonadotrophin-releasing hormone analogues for endometriosis. *Drug Therap Bull* 1993; 31: 21–2.

6   Matta WH, Shaw RW, Hesp R, Evans R. Reversible trabecular bone density loss following induced hypo-oestrogenism with the GnRH analogue, buserelin, in premenopausal women. *Clin Endocrinol* 1988; 29: 45–51.

7   Prentice A, Deary AJ, Goldbeck-Wood S, Farquhar C, Smith SK. Gonadotrophin-releasing hormone analogues for pain associated with endometriosis. *Cochrane Database Syst Rev* 1999; (1).

8   Howell R, Edmonds DK, Dowsett M, Crook D, Lees B, Stevenson JC. Gonadotrophin-releasing hormone analogue (goserelin) plus hormone replacement therapy for the treatment of endometriosis: a randomised controlled trial. *Fertil Steril* 1995; 64: 474–81.

9   Moghissi KS, Schlaff WD, Olive DL, Skinner MA, Yin H. Goserelin acetate (Zoladex) with or without hormone replacement therapy for the treatment of endometriosis. *Fertil Steril* 1998; 69: 1056–62.

10 Compston JE, Yamaguchi K, Groucher PI, Garrahan NJ, Lindsay PC, Shaw RW. The effects of gonadotrophin-releasing hormone agonists on iliac crest cancellous bone structure in women with endometriosis. *Bone* 1995; 16: 261–7.

11 Lindsay PC, Shaw RW, Bennink HJC, Kicovic P. The effect of add-back treatment with tibolone (Livial) on patients treated with the gonadotrophin-releasing hormone agonist triptorelin (De-capeptyl). *Fertil Steril* 1996; 65: 342–8.

12 Taskin O, Yalcinoglu AI, Kucuk S, Uryan I, Buhur A, Burak F. Effectiveness of tibolone on hypoestrogenic symptoms induced by goserelin treatment in patients with endometriosis. *Fertil Steril* 1997; 67: 40–5.

13 Gregoriou O, Konidaris S, Vitoratos N, Papadias C, Papoulias I, Chryssicopoulos A. Gonadotrophin-releasing hormone analogue plus hormone replacement therapy for the treatment of endometriosis: a randomised controlled trial. *Int J Fertil* 1997; 42: 406–11.

14 Fedele L, Bianchi S, Zanconato G, Portuese A, Raffaelli R. Use of levonorgestrel-releasing intrauterine device in the treatment of rectovaginal endometriosis. *Fertil Steril* 2001; 75: 485–488.

15 Bulun SE, Zeitoun K, Takayama K, Noble L, Michael D, Simpson E, Johns A, Putman M, Sasano H. Estrogen production in endometriosis and use of aromatase inhibitors to treat endometriosis. *Endocrine related cancer* 1999; 6: 293–301.

16 Bulun SE, Zeitoun K, Takayama K, Sasano H. Molecular basis for treating endometriosis with aromatase inhibitors. *Hum Reprod* 2000; 6: 413–418.

17 Telimaa S, Puolakka J, Ronnberg L, Kauppila A. Placebo-controlled comparison of danazol and high-dose medroxyprogesterone acetate in the treatment of endometriosis. *Gynecol Endocrinol* 1987; 1: 13–23.

18 Dlugi AM, Miller JD, Knittle J, and the Lupron Study Group. Lupron depot (leuprolide acetate for depot suspension) in the treatment of endometriosis: a randomised, placebo-controlled, double-blind study. *Fertil Steril* 1990: 54: 419–27.

19 Ling FW. Randomised controlled trial of depot leuprolide in patients with chronic pelvic pain and clinically suspected endometriosis. *Obstet Gynecol* 1999; 93: 51–8.

20 Overton CE, Lindsay PC, Johal B, Collins SA, Siddle NC, Shaw RW, Barlow DH. A randomised, double-blind, placebo-controlled study of luteal phase dydrogesterone (Duphaston) in women with minimal to mild endometriosis. *Fertil Steril* 1994; 62: 701–7.

21 Moore J, Kennedy S, Prentice A. Modern combined oral contraceptives for pain associated with endometriosis (Cochrane Review). The Cochrane Database Syst Rev, 1999; (1).

22 Vercellini P, Trespidi L, Colombo A, Vendola N, Marchini M, Crosignani PG. A gonadotrophin-releasing hormone agonist versus a low-dose oral contraceptive for pelvic pain associated with endometriosis. *Fertil Steril* 1993; 60: 75–9.

23 Fedele L, Bianchi S, Viezzoli T, Arcaini L, Candiani GB. Gestrinone versus danazol in the treatment of endometriosis. *Fertil Steril* 1989; 51: 781–5.

24 The Gestrinone Italian Study Group. Gestrinone versus a gonadotrophin-releasing hormone agonist for the treatment of pelvic pain associated with endometriosis: a multicenter, randomised, double-blind study. *Fertil Steril* 1996; 66: 911–9.

25 Hughes E, Fedorkow D, Collins J, Vandekerckhove P. Ovulation suppression for endometriosis (Cochrane Review). The Cochrane Database Syst Rev, 1999; (1).

26 Crikel U, Ochs H, Schneider HP. A randomised comparative trial of triptorelin depot (D-Trp6-LHRH) and danazol in the treatment of endometriosis. *Eur J Obstet Gynaecol Reprod Biol* 1995; 59: 61–9.

27 Dmowski WP, Tummon I, Pepping P, Radwanska E, Binor Z. Ovarian suppression induced with buserelin or danazol in the management of endometriosis: a randomised comparative study. *Fertil Steril* 1989; 51: 395–400.

28 Rana N, Thomas S, Rotman C, Dmowski WP. Decrease in the size of ovarian endometriomas during ovarian suppression in Stage IV endometriosis. Role of preoperative medical treatment. *J Reprod Med* 1996; 41: 384–92.

29 Donnez J, Nisolle-Pochet M, Clerckx-Braun F, Sandow J, Casanas-Roux F. Administration of nasal buserelin as compared with subcutaneous buserelin implant for endometriosis. *Fertil Steril* 1989; 52: 27–30.

30 Parazzini F, Fedele L, Busacca M et al. Postsurgical medical treatment of advanced endometriosis: results of a randomised clinical trial. *Am J Obstet Gynecol* 1994; 171: 1205–7.

31 Hornstein MD, Hemmings R, Yuzpe AA, Heinrichs WL. Use of nafarelin versus placebo after reductive laparoscopic surgery for endometriosis. *Fertil Steril* 1997; 68: 860–4

CHAPTER 5

Surgical treatment

Laparoscopic surgery

In the pioneering days of operative laparoscopy, the Frenchman, Raoul Palmer, and the German, Hans Frangenheim, popularised laparoscopic surgery, but it was essentially limited in its use to female sterilisation and the aspiration and fenestration of ovarian cysts. Kurt Semm, a trained engineer as well as a brilliant surgeon, took operative laparoscopy one stage further. He invented several instruments and techniques that were necessary for the keyhole approach,[1] and he described a series of operations that could be performed safely through small incisions avoiding the complication of a large laparotomy incision.[2]

At that time, electrosurgery had been associated with a large number of accidents during the performance of female sterilisation, which were due to a stray radio-frequency current inherent in early electrosurgical generators. The frustration at being unable to cut and coagulate effectively with electrosurgery quickly led to the early enthusiasm for laparoscopic laser surgery.[3–6]

Advantages of laparoscopic surgery

Laparoscopic surgery embraces all the principles of microsurgery:

- adequate exposure
- magnification

- minimal tissue handlin
- strict attention to haemostasi
- prevention of tissue desiccation.

The pneumoperitoneum inflates the abdomen and keeps the bowel out of the operation site, ensuring adequate exposure and an excellent view. The magnification factor of a laparoscope is around eight-fold. The use of lasers ensures a non-contact method of operating, so there is minimal tissue handling, and strict attention is paid to haemostasis. Frequent irrigation with warm heparinised Ringer-Lactate solution, used to prevent fogging of the laparoscope and to clear away any blood or debris, also prevents tissue desiccation, which is a potent cause of adhesion formation. Additionally, laparoscopic surgery reduces the risk of infection because of the closed environment and non-contact method of surgery. The minimal access (or keyhole) approach results in several small and less painful scars. These benefits are reflected in a much shorter hospital stay, and most patients can be operated on in a daycare setting. The smaller scars inevitably mean a quicker return to full activity for the woman:

- reduced infection risk
- less painful scars
- shorter hospital stay
- quicker return to full activity
- less postoperative adhesion formation.

Avoidance of adhesions

Laparoscopic surgery in experimental animals has been shown to result in less adhesion formation,[7] and this is believed to be due, in part, to the decreased handling of tissues and the copious use of irrigant fluids. Since most adhesions form within

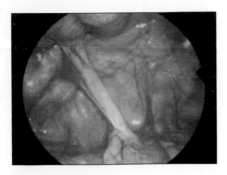

Figure 5.1 *Adhesions due to endometriosis*

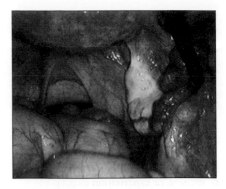

Figure 5.2 *Methylene blue dye spilling from the right fallopian tube to confirm tubal patency*

the first few hours of surgery[8] and are the direct result of a peritoneal insult, a volume of fluid (0.5–1.0 litres) is left *in situ* at the end of most laparoscopic surgical procedures, in order to avoid adhesion formation[9] (Figure 5.1).

The minimal handling of tissue in laparoscopic surgery and the absence of packs to contain the bowel result in less peritoneal trauma, while the avoidance of sutures results in less tissue ischaemia.[10]

Newer anti-adhesion barrier solutions, such as 4% icodextrin, which has been used in peritoneal dialysis for many years, are employed to create a fluid barrier between the healing surfaces and can remain in the peritoneal cavity for up to seven days. Patients are aware of a slightly unpleasant feeling of fluid moving around inside the abdominal cavity and can experience an exacerbation of the shoulder tip pain, which is quite common after laparoscopic surgery. Occasionally, fluid may leak out through the small skin incisions. If the fluid leaks beneath the skin surface, it is rapidly broken down by amylase in the subcutaneous tissues, and any leakage merely needs to be treated by the application of waterproof plasters until it ceases.

Less chance of recurrent disease

The advent of laparoscopic surgery occurred at a time when physicians were becoming increasingly disillusioned with medical treatment approaches to endometriosis. In many instances, the disease was suppressed by the medication but recurred after cessation of treatment.[11] Additionally, the drugs were ineffective against ovarian endometriomas and deeply infiltrating disease in the rectovaginal septum, which appeared to be increasingly common. A paper by Waller and Shaw[12] showed that there was a disease recurrence rate of 53.4% at five years of follow-up, whereas long-term follow-up after surgical excision at laparoscopy showed only 19% recurrence at five years.[13]

Aims of conservative surgery in laparoscopy

Most women presenting with symptoms of endometriosis do so at a relatively early age and conservative surgery is therefore essential in order to retain their potential for fertility. Some women do not present with symptoms of pain, but the endometriosis is discovered during the work-up for infertility, when a diagnostic laparoscopy and dye test is performed (Figure 5.2). The aims of conservative surgery are:

- cytoreduction of ectopic endometrial tissue
- restoration of normal tubo-ovarian anatomy
- interruption of afferent sensory pathways
- removal of ovarian endometriomas
- excision or vaporisation of deep infiltrating disease in the uterosacral ligaments, pelvic side wall and rectovaginal septum.

All ectopic endometrial tissue is either vaporised with the laser or excised by electrosurgery or with the ultrasonic scalpel. This means the removal of the black deposits of haemosiderin; the red flame-like lesions, with their associated neoangiogenesis that implies active implants; all the vesicular lesions (sago grains); the yellow-brown lesions on the peritoneal surface; and any white infiltrating disease, which usually signifies fibromuscular hyperplasia around ectopic endometrial glands and stroma. In advanced disease, it is important to restore the normal tubo-ovarian anatomy by dividing any adhesions caused by the

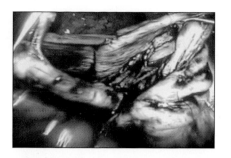

Figure 5.3 *Excision of an endometrioma*

endometriosis, to enable the Fallopian tube to pick up and transport the oocyte effectively. This is particularly important when the tubes are grossly distorted and swollen as they course over a large ovarian endometrioma. This necessitates freeing the endometrioma from the pelvic sidewall, which usually results in the release of old haemosiderin ('chocolate fluid') that is aspirated and the site irrigated until the effluent runs clear, and then the lining of the endometrioma is either excised (Figure 5.3) or vaporised with a laser or bipolar coagulation (Figures 5.4a & b).

Many of these laparoscopic surgical procedures involve the interruption of afferent sensory pathways, either by uterine nerve ablation or by presacral neurectomy, to decrease dysmenorrhoea, the leading

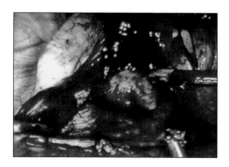

Figure 5.4(a) *An endometrioma being opened prior to coagulation of the cyst wall with an electosurgical diathermy*

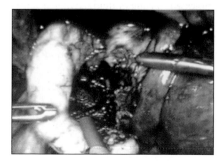

Figure 5.4(b) *Endometrioma following coagulation of the cyst wall*

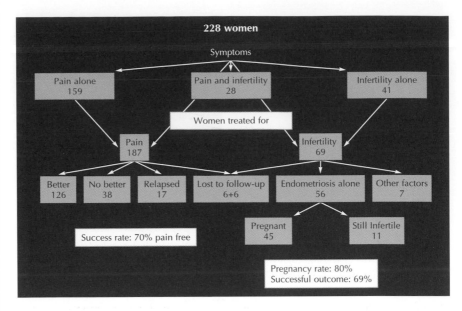

Figure 5.5 *Results of laser laparoscopy in women with endometriosis (with permission)*

presenting symptom of many patients with endometriosis. The role of these denervation procedures is still controversial and will be dealt with later.

Laser laparoscopy

Early developments

During the 1980s, centres in Europe and the USA reported the effectiveness of various lasers in relieving the pain of endometriosis in 60–70% of women with the carbon dioxide (CO_2) laser.[14–16] Similar results were achieved with the neodymium:YAG laser,[17] the argon laser[18] and the KTP/532 laser.[19]

When we started using the CO_2 laser via the laparoscope in 1982, we were mainly concerned with the safety of using such a high-powered energy source within the abdominal cavity. In fact, it turned out to be very safe: during the last 18 years,

having treated over 12 500 women, we have had no accidents with the CO_2 laser.

Our next important goal was to look at the effectiveness of using the laser to ablate peritoneal endometriosis. We therefore followed our first 228 patients over five years (Figure 5.5) and, at the end of that time, 126 of the 187 women suffering from pain (70%) were pain-free.

Thirty-eight of these women experienced no improvement, and most were subjected to a second-look procedure, which failed to reveal any sign of recurrent endometriosis. It was subsequently discovered that many of these women had different reasons for their pelvic pain, including irritable bowel syndrome and various psychological problems (two women were diagnosed as having Münchausen syndrome).

Seventeen women suffered a relapse during the five-year follow-up and second-look laparoscopy showed that endometriosis had recurred, but almost always at different sites. Six women were lost to follow-up. Of the 56 patients with infertility due to endometriosis alone, 45 became pregnant, giving an 80% pregnancy rate.[16]

Unfortunately, this study was performed retrospectively and, although it is difficult to argue with the recorded conception rates, recording the relief of pain – a highly subjective phenomenon – is a different matter. It would be entirely possible for a surgeon to influence the result of the pain relief, particularly when using highly technological equipment such as a laser, which tends to increase a patient's perception of the efficacy of the operation, and in some instances, the patient will indicate that pain relief has been achieved in order to please the surgeon.

The only way to resolve this issue is to perform a prospective, double-blind, randomised, controlled trial, so that neither the patient nor the person following up the patient is aware of whether the intervention is merely a diagnostic laparoscopy alone or includes laser surgery. In 1994, we published the results of such a trial, which remains the first and, to our knowledge, only such trial on endometriosis reported in the world literature.[20]

The Guildford laser laparoscopy trial

Background
The aim of this study,[20] which was undertaken at our unit in Guildford, UK, in women suffering from minimal to moderate endometriosis (AFS stages I–III), was to assess the efficacy of laser laparoscopy by comparing the results of those who received laser treatment with

the results of those who underwent diagnostic laparo-scopy only.[21] The study was approved by the hospital ethics committee, but only for patients up to AFS stage III. It was felt to be unethical to withhold laser treatment from women in severe pain due to stage IV disease, chiefly because our previous experience had shown 80% pain relief in this patient group, the majority of whom had failed to respond to medical therapy.[22]

The study population was recruited from women seen in the gynaecological outpatient clinic, who were experiencing pain suggestive of endometriosis and who had been advised to undergo a diagnostic laparoscopy. Prior to laparoscopy, the women were asked to record the intensity of their pain on a 10-cm, linear analogue scale, marked from 0 (no pain at all) to 10 (worst pain the woman had experienced in her life).[23]

Between March 1990 and February 1993, 74 women were recruited and, at the time of laparoscopy treatment, randomly allocated to either the laser-treatment or the expectant-management group, using a computer-generated randomisation sequence. The laser treatment included vaporisation of all visible endometriotic implants, adhesiolysis and uterine nerve transection using a triple puncture technique. The patients in the sham arm received exactly the same incisions but merely had a diagnostic laparoscopy, although it was necessary to remove the serosanguinous fluid from the pouch of Douglas in order to perform a thorough inspection of the entire pelvic peritoneum. Patients were not informed of which treatment group they had been allocated to and were followed up at three and six

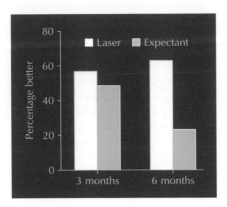

Figure 5.6 *Proportion of women with pain symptom alleviation at all stages (with permission)*

months after surgery by an independent observer (research nurse), who was unaware of which treatment had been allocated.

Results of the trial

Of 74 women who entered the trial, 63 (32 from the laser-treated arm and 31 from the expectant-management arm) completed the study to the point of the six-month follow-up visit. The 11 women no longer in the trial were excluded because eight had either become pregnant or been prescribed the oral contraceptive pill (despite requests to the patients and to their doctors not to do so during the course of the trial), and three were lost to follow-up. The trial results are shown in Figures 5.6 and 5.7, and it can be seen clearly that, at three months following the operation, there was very little difference between the two groups whereas, at six months, the difference reached statistical significance, with 62.5% of the laser-treatment patients showing improvement compared with only 22.6% of the sham group. The results were least convincing for stage I disease, and this is probably because some of the minimal

changes seen in mild endometriosis could possibly be due to inflammatory changes, or Walthard's cell rests, or other non-specific changes in the peritoneum. Disease confirmation by biopsy was not permitted, because taking a biopsy can be interpreted as a cyto-reductive procedure and therefore cannot be part of true expectant management. If stage I patients were excluded from the analysis, 73.7% of patients achieved pain relief, which is very similar to the figure obtained in our retrospective study.[16]

Lessons learned from the Guildford laser laparoscopy trial

There are several interesting features of this study that merit discussion. We were surprised that the results at three months were very similar for the laser-treated group (56%) and the expectant-management group (48%). There was no significant difference between these two figures and we were surprised to find that almost half of the women with no treatment claimed to feel better. This placebo effect has been noticed in other studies, where dysmenorrhoea was reported to have improved in up to 30% of women in the placebo arm

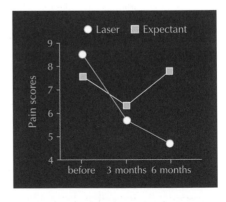

Figure 5.7 *Median visual analogue pain scores (with time) (with permission)*

of an Italian study comparing expectant management with GnRH analogues.[24] The improvement noted in the placebo arm did not last longer than three months, mirroring our findings exactly. The visual analogue scale used in our study shows particularly clearly that, at six months following laparoscopy, expectant-management patients had returned to the original score, whereas laser-treated patients had continued to improve. Thus, it may take at least three months for the benefit of laparoscopic laser surgery to be noticed, and we now advise patients of this and only see them for follow-up at six months.

Another benefit of this trial was that it allowed us to look at the natural history of endometriosis, generally assumed to be a progressive disease. We had the opportunity to investigate a group of women who had not received any treatment but had an established diagnosis, and to report the findings of the second-look laparoscopy alongside changes in their symptoms.[25] At second-look laparoscopy, ten cases (42%) showed no change in he AFS score; seven cases (29%) had an increased score, with three women moving to a higher stage, and, to our surprise, one-third of the women (seven cases) had a reduced AFS score, with three moving to a lower stage. These women had improved or resolved symptoms, whereas the symptomatology in the other women had remained the same or become more severe, while waiting for laparo-scopic laser surgery. We were able to show that the disease is progressive in the majority of cases but, in up to one-third of women, it can regress or (rarely) disappeared altogether. This finding has also been confirmed in studies on experimentally induced endometriosis in higher primates.[26]

Long-term follow-up of the women in the trial

We have now conducted a long-term follow-up of the cohort of women who underwent laser laparoscopy in the initial trial.[27] Of 56 laser-treated women, 38 (67.9%) were contacted successfully; the remaining women (44.6%) had been lost to follow-up after three years. The mean time since operation was 73 months. The mean age of women was 37 years (range, 27–50 years) compared with 27 years (range, 19–41 years) at the time of surgery. The recurrence of painful symptoms had occurred in 28 (73.7%) women at some point since their operation. The median time for recurrence was 19.7 months (range, 5–60 months).

At the time of follow-up, satisfactory symptom relief had occurred in 21 (55.3%) patients. One woman was menopausal and seven were leading pain-free lives, none having had need of further intervention. Two women had undergone hysterectomy and endometriosis was found at operation. Repeat laser laparoscopies to treat new endometriosis were performed in eight women. Medical therapy was being used successfully to control mild symptoms in three women.

Of the remaining 17 (44.7%) women, who continued to experience painful symptoms, 11 had undergone further surgery on one or more occasion. Eight of these women had eventually had a hysterectomy and were noted to have a normal pelvis at operation. Repeat laser laparoscopies to treat new endometriosis were performed in two patients. A further two women were receiving psychiatric care in combination with analgesic medication, and one woman was in an assisted-conception programme. Medical therapy was being used to control

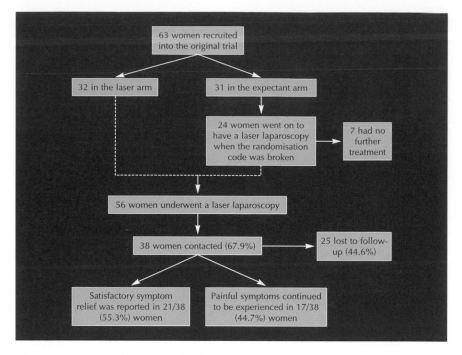

Figure 5.8 *Long-term follow-up results of women who underwent laser laparoscopy in the treatment of pelvic pain associated with minimal to moderate endometriosis (with permission)*

severe symptoms in two patients; one patient complained of pain but was not being treated for it (Figure 5.8).

Pelvic denervation procedures

Since pelvic pain and dysmenorrhoea are common symptoms among young women, it is not surprising that many attempts have been made to interrupt some of the afferent sensory nerve fibres supplying the uterus. The operation of presacral neurectomy by laparotomy has a long history and was first described in the 1930s.[28] In those days, it was a formidable operation with a relatively high complication rate and a failure rate of around 11–15% in primary dysmenorrhoea and 25–40% in secondary dysmenorrhoea, mainly due to endometriosis.[29,30]

In 1954, Doyle described the procedure of paracervical uterine denervation, which bears his name.[31] Doyle's procedure involved the excision of the uterosacral ligaments, which carry most of the sensory pain fibres to the lower part of the uterus, at their attachment to the posterior aspect of the cervix. He suggested that the procedure could be performed vaginally by gynaecologists, but that general surgeons might prefer a large laparotomy incision. His results were extremely impressive, with complete pain relief in 63 of 73 women (86%), partial pain relief in six cases, and only four failures. With such a satisfactory outcome it is difficult to see why the operation sank into obscurity, but possibly this was due to the advent of the oral contraceptive pill and prostaglandin synthetase inhibitors, which reduced the demand for such relatively drastic forms of surgical intervention. However, interest in Doyle's procedure has been revived with the advent of minimal access surgery. Laparoscopic uterine nerve ablation (LUNA) takes only a few minutes to perform with a surgical laser or electro-surgical needle and it produces the same tissue effect without the need for major surgery and with an extremely low complication rate.

Anatomy of the uterine nerve supply

The perfect neuro-ablative surgical procedure for pelvic pain would interrupt all the afferent sensory nerves from all the pelvic organs and leave all other nerves unaffected. Unfortunately, this is not possible because the uterus and the ovaries receive their nerve supply not only through a series of nervous plexuses, but also by nerves that accompany the ovarian and uterine arteries. The diagram in Figure 5.9 shows that it would be impossible to interrupt all these nervous pathways without damaging the vascular supply of the reproductive organs.[32]

The body of the uterus appears to be innervated only by sympathetic fibres[33] The cervix is mainly supplied by para-sympathetic fibres that traverse the cervical division of the Lee–Frankenhauser plexus,

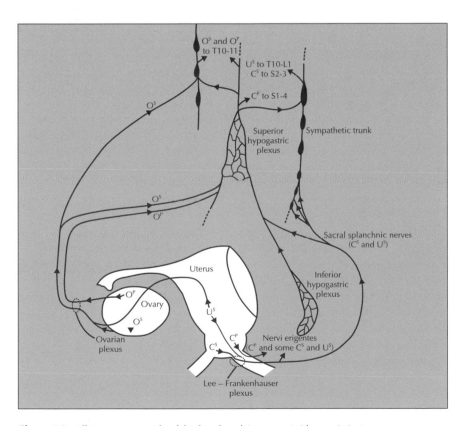

Figure 5.9 *Afferent nerve supply of the female pelvic organs (with permission)*

which lies in, under and around the attachments of the uterosacral ligament to the posterolateral aspect of the cervix.[34-36] Sympathetic fibres can also be found in this area, which have reached the cervix by accompanying the uterine arteries. Excellent illustrations of Lee's dissection showing the nerves in this plexus can be seen in the Wellcome Historical Museum, London, UK.

From the uterosacral ligaments, the parasympathetic afferent fibres reach the dorsal root ganglia of the first to fourth sacral spinal nerves (S1-4) via the pelvic splanchnic nerves (nervi erigentes) and the inferior hypogastric plexus. Theoretically, therefore, division of the uterosacral ligaments at the point of their attachment to the cervix should result in the interruption of most of the cervical sensory fibres and some of the corporal sensory fibres, leading to a diminution in uterine pain at the time of menstruation. However, it is clear that the sympathetic afferent fibres that accompany the uterine, iliac, and inferior mesenteric arteries to the sacral sympathetic trunk via the sacral splanchnic nerves will not be interrupted, rendering complete denervation impossible.

Surgical division of the uterosacral ligaments by LUNA or resection of the presacral nerves can be expected to diminish central pain from dysmenorrhoea with reasonable certainty. However, they cannot be expected to relieve lateral pain, especially that coming from the ovaries, because the relevant nerve fibres bypass the uterosacral ligament and course through the corresponding plexuses to their cells of origin in the dorsal route ganglia of the tenth and eleventh thoracic spinal nerves. Indeed, some of the afferent nerves of the upper ovarian plexus run directly via the renal and aortic plexuses and also bypass the superior hyporgastric plexus, so that even a complete presacral neurectomy would not interrupt them.

Laparoscopic uterine nerve ablation

In women with either primary or secondary dysmenorrhoea, LUNA can be performed at the same time as a diag-nostic laparoscopy. The pelvis should be inspected carefully for associated pathology, particularly endometriosis. If this is found, the endometriotic implants should be vaporised using a CO_2 laser or removed by electrosurgery. The broad ligaments should be inspected carefully, to try to identify the course of the ureter, and the ligaments are vaporised forming a crater of about 2-cm in diameter and 1-cm in depth. The procedure should continue until all the nerve fibres have been divided. Sometimes, in advanced endometriosis, the uterosacral ligaments are infiltrated with endometrial glands and stroma and the surrounding fibromuscular hyperplasia, and it is possible that the removal of all this disease tissue is an important contributing factor to the good results of this procedure. Our group has been performing this operation for 18 years and we have had no cases of mortality or serious morbidity. However, there have been reports in the world literature of two deaths from secondary haemorrhage[37] and of two cases of subsequent prolapse, but this is almost certainly coincidental because the uterosacral ligaments do not play a major part in pelvic floor support.[38]

Presacral neurectomy

The operation of presacral neurectomy at laparotomy has been in use for at least

70 years, and the first published series was in 1937.[28] Because of the relatively high incidence of complications, this type of major abdominal surgery is rarely used nowadays, although in the hands of an extremely experienced, skilled laparoscopic surgeon, it can be performed laparoscopically even on a daycare basis. It is a highly difficult laparoscopic procedure because the retroperitoneal space in front of the sacral promontory is extremely vascular, with widely varying anatomical configurations.[39] It is necessary to deflect the sigmoid colon laterally, aided by a left-sided tilt of the operating table, and to be absolutely certain of obtaining haemostasis before dividing or excising the nerves of the superior hypogastric plexus. There have been reports that the beam of some devices, such as the argon-beam coagulator, has reflected off the surface of the periosteum, tearing the common iliac vessels and leading to catastrophic bleeding.[40] However, in skilled hands, the operation will offer good long-term results.[41,42]

Unfortunately, this procedure has a high incidence of complications; for example, in a study by Chen et al.,[47] 31 of 33 patients who underwent laparoscopic presacral neurectomy experienced constipation, which was very severe in some cases. In another study on presacral neurectomy at laparotomy, Candiani et al.[43] reported that 13 women had long-standing constipation, three had urinary urgency and two had a completely asymptomatic first stage of labour. There was also one woman who required a subsequent laparotomy 48 hours postoperatively because of a presacral haematoma.

Laparoscopic presacral neurectomy is regarded as being an extremely advanced level IV procedure, to be performed exclusively in highly specialised centres. Laparoscopic uterine nerve ablation, on the other hand, should be within the skill of any reasonably competent laparoscopic surgery unit as found in most district general hospitals. Unfortunately, however, two recent randomised collaborative trials[44,45] have cast some doubt on the efficacy of these denervation procedures. This will be dealt with in the final section of this chapter.

Fertility-enhancing procedures

There is little doubt that a woman with one or two large ovarian endometriomas, or 'chocolate cysts', will be subfertile because of the gross distortion of the fallopian tube as it is stretched over the enlarged ovary, making ovum pick-up virtually impossible. Nevertheless, the fimbrial ends are usually quite healthy and the tubes patent, with no functional abnormality. Thus, once the large ovary is returned to a normal size and the adhesions are divided surgically, dye used to check the patency of the tube will spill promptly through the healthy fimbrial ends and a good pregnancy will rate follow. In our initial study of 106 women, we reported a pregnancy rate of 57%, most of these patients becoming pregnant within six to nine months of the procedure.[46] When we formally published this study a little later, it included 165 women treated with either the CO_2 laser or the KTP laser, and we found that the efficacy of the CO_2 laser was less than that of the KTP laser. This was due to the fact that the former is almost totally absorbed by water molecules and, therefore, cannot be expected to work as well in the presence of the old blood, which is the 'chocolate fluid' inside the endometrioma. Even when restricting the data analysis to those women treated with the KTP laser, the pregnancy rate was 47.6%. The probable reason for this decreased rate was that our clinical unit had then become a tertiary referral centre and the patient population shifted towards those who had had previous surgery, previous failed attempts at *in vitro* fertilisation, and very large endometriomas[47] Nevertheless, against a background pregnancy rate of zero in women with severe disease, this is an extremely good pregnancy rate and much higher than that achieved with assisted conception.[48]

Some authorities have suggested that the relationship of mild endometriosis with infertility is casual rather than causal,[49] so that the discovery of a few peritoneal deposits of endometriosis may just be a chance finding and not actually be implicated in the aetiology of the disease. It is well known that many women with minimal or mild endometriosis will get pregnant without intervention, although several studies have shown that their monthly fecundity rate is much lower than that of the general population.[48,50] The real problem in assessing treatment efficacy in mild or minimal endometriosis lies in establishing whether any form of treatment has a clear advantage over the mere act of tubal insufflation with methylene blue dye and the aspiration of the yellow serosanguinous fluid from the pouch of Douglas, which is known to be laden with activated macrophages, interleukins, other cytokines, and prostanoids.[51] Using these simple techniques, one can expect an overall pregnancy rate of 50.3% (range, 30.6–72.4%) in women with mild endometriosis[48,52] It is important to realise, however, that these studies referred to mild disease exclusively, and the only report of

expectant management in moderate disease (stage III) gave a corrected pregnancy rate of merely 25% and there were no conceptions at all in women with severe disease (stage IV).[48]

We have little doubt that laparoscopic laser surgery has a beneficial effect with regard to an increase in pregnancy rates. Because restoration of the tubo-ovarian anatomy is so important for women with stage IV disease, it is not surprising that our best results have been attained in women with advanced-stage endometriosis. The 80% pregnancy rate achieved in our five-year study in women with no other infertility factors is impressive.[16] Our data compare favourably with publications from the USA[53] and Europe,[6,54] which reflect early work with laser laparoscopy in several centres in the late 1980s.

All the initial studies were retrospective and, thus, inherently prone to the possible misinterpretation of facts; an example would be counting a pregnancy as a success, when actually the woman was not intending to conceive. It is, therefore, essential to demand good, evidence-based science in the form of randomised, prospective, controlled studies, before accepting the efficacy of a new form of treatment. In an unpublished trial fulfilling these criteria, we recruited 27 patients, 14 of whom had laser laparoscopic removal of any active endometriotic lesions and their associated adhesions, while 13 merely had any fluid removed that had accumulated in the pouch of Douglas; dye was passed through the tubes to check for patency in both groups. At the end of one year, 50% of women in the laser-treated group had become pregnant, whereas half that number in the no-treatment group had conceived. The pregnancy rate in the no-treatment group was virtually identical to those found in two other controlled studies where medical treatment was compared to placebo placebo.[55,56]

There are two published, randomised, controlled trials comparing diagnostic laparoscopy alone to surgical ablation of minimal to mild endometriosis. The Endocam Study[44] recruited 341 women who were undergoing diagnostic laparoscopy and who were found to have minimal or mild endometriosis. It involved 25 fertility clinics throughout Canada. Randomisation was performed at the time of diagnostic laparoscopy, and it was necessary to telephone a number, manned 24 hours a day, in order to ascertain whether the woman was to undergo resection or ablation of visible endometriosis and adhesions or to undergo diagnostic laparoscopy and hydrotubation alone. The women were followed for 36 weeks after laparoscopy or, in the case of those who became pregnant during that interval, for up to 20 weeks of pregnancy. Among the 172 women who had resection or ablation of the endo-metriosis, 50 became pregnant and had pregnancies that continued for 20 weeks or longer, compared with only 29 of the 169 women in the diagnostic-laparoscopy group (cumulative probabilities, 30.7% and 17.7%, respectively; P = 0.006). The corresponding rates of fecundity were 4.7 and 2.4 per 100 person months (rate ratio, 1.9; 95% confidence interval, 1.2–3.1).

In a smaller study by Parazzini,[45] ten out of 51 women (19.6%) in the treatment group, as opposed to ten out of 45 women (22.2%) in the control group, became pregnant within one year following laparoscopy, suggesting no intergroup difference.

Deeply infiltrating endometriosis

Deeply infiltrating endometriosis is almost invariably located in the rectovaginal septum or the uterosacral ligaments and is sometimes found in the uterovesical fold – in areas composed of muscle and fibrous connective tissue. This nodular or fibrous tissue can be felt, rather than seen, and is particularly painful around the time of menstruation. In some women, no endometriosis can be seen laparoscopically, but the induration can be felt clearly by a combination of rectal and vaginal examination. These spherical endometriotic nodules in the rectovaginal septum can be clearly felt as painful nodules at that site, and colposcopic examination of the vagina often reveals dark blue domed cysts, about 3–4 mm in diameter, in the posterior vaginal fornix. These are the most severe lesions and have a tendency to spread laterally up and around the uterine artery and sometimes cause sclerosis around the ureter, although, interestingly, they never appear to invade the layers of the ureteric wall. The behaviour of this type of deeply infiltrating disease, which is virtually unresponsive to drug therapy, is such that it can be considered an indirect argument for the hypothesis that deep endometriosis has escaped from the inhibitory influence of the peritoneal fluid and is mainly under the control of the peripheral circulation.[57]

Possible environmental aetiological factors

Koninckx *et al.*[58] have suggested that dioxin and polychlorinated-biphenyl pollution is a possible cofactor in the cause and development of deeply infiltrating endometriosis, which may be contributing to the steadily increasing number of hysterectomies that are being performed.[59] Epidemiological data reported by the World Health Organisation show the highest concentrations of dioxin in breast milk to be in Belgium,[60] which also appears to be the country with the highest incidence of endometriosis in the world, and much of this is of the deeply infiltrating type.[61] The highest concentration of cases within Belgium is found in the industrial corridor running along the south of the country (Donnez J, personal communication).

Dioxin has immunosuppressive activities and is a potent inhibitor of T-lymphocyte function.[62,63] Rhesus monkeys that were chronically exposed to dioxin for a period of four years were found to develop endometriosis seven years after the termination of dioxin exposure, and in the majority of cases, the disease was of the deeply infiltrating variety.[8] Dioxin is a potentially harmful byproduct of the chlorine-bleaching process used in the wood pulp industry, which includes the manufacture of feminine hygiene products such as tampons. This may chronically expose the rectovaginal septum and posterior fornix to a known immunosuppressant.

Surgical treatment

Laparoscopic inspection, ultrasonography, or MRI are not completely adequate to delineate these deeply infiltrating lesions. This can only be done properly during surgical excision and subsequent pathological inspection to determine the lesion's shape and depth of penetration. Before any operative laparoscopy is performed, the woman should have a proctoscopy and sigmoidoscopy, preferably during menst-

ruation in addition to any appropriate radiological investigations. In the case of the lesion extending laterally, an intravenous urogram is required but, if the lesion is confined to the rectovaginal septum it is our practice to perform an air-contrast barium enema, sometimes combined with a vaginogram, which should be carefully examined in the lateral views. A thorough bowel preparation is mandatory in all women suspected of having deep endometriosis, and women should be warned that there is a real risk of perforating the bowel. If this does happen, a colorectal surgeon should be on hand to repair such a defect. However, if the bowel preparation has been satisfactory, a colostomy should not be necessary and some of the perforations can be repaired adequately transanally or even laparoscopically.[65]

In the past, it has been necessary to resort to laparotomy for women with deeply infiltrating endometriosis, but with increased experience in laparoscopic surgery, many of them can be treated by laparoscopy using CO_2 laser or elecro-surgical excision, or sharp dissection with scissors. In addition, it is sometimes necessary to perform vaginal excision, either from below or by laparoscopy, once the plane of cleavage has been developed between the rectum and the vagina.[65–68] Inevitably with this kind of surgery, which is probably the most difficult type of laparoscopic surgery requiring considerable skill and experience, each surgeon will use the method that is best suited to them. In our department, we use a high-power superpulse CO_2 laser to develop the plane of cleavage between the rectum and the vagina, with special instrumentation to separate these two structures from below and careful palpation to avoid damaging the rectum.

Even in highly skilled hands, bowel perforation happens from time to time, and Nezhat et al.[68] reported a series of 174 women in which nine women suffered bowel perforations and a further two required ureteric stents. Nevertheless, moderate or complete pain relief was achieved in 162 of the women. If dissection has to be very close to the rectum, it is a wise precaution to fill the pelvis with warm Ringer-Lactate solution and insufflate the rectum with air or methylene blue dye to look for any unrecognised rectal lacerations or perforations.[65] A vaginal incision is often, but not routinely, required and when the vagina is opened, the procedure may be completed vaginally or laparoscopically. In addition, it is sometimes possible to vaporise the vaginal blue domed cysts via a colposcope, with a finger inserted in the rectum to make sure that the vaporisation does not damage the rectum.

To excise uterosacral nodules, the peritoneum is incised lateral to the uterosacral ligament. It is necessary to first identify the ureter and, occasionally, to dissect it out along its course. Once it is displaced laterally, the uterosacral ligament is resected beginning posteriorly and working towards the uterus. Once the nodule has been freed from the underlying tissue, the anterior part of the ligament is cut and most of these deep uterosacral implants can be treated without any need for a vaginal incision.

Women with full-thickness bowel or bladder lesions require more extensive surgery, which is probably better dealt with by laparotomy, although some very advanced laparoscopic surgeons have reported successful results employing transanal circular stapling devices[65] and laparoscopic and transanal or transvaginal repair with or without the help of colorectal surgeons.[69,70]

Although this type of surgery is difficult and time consuming, the results justify the effort, particularly since many of these patients are unresponsive to medical therapy. Koninckx and Martin analysed their results in 250 women, in whom deep endometriosis had been excised with the CO_2 laser, and showed a cure rate of pelvic pain of 70%, with a recurrence rate of less than 5% within a follow-up period of up to five years.[57] These results should be interpreted bearing in mind that there is always a learning curve in this kind of surgery. Closer inspection of the data reveals that the completeness of excision steadily increased with experience, and the results of the more recent years strongly suggest an almost complete cure rate with a very low recurrence rate.

A critical appraisal of the evidence for neuroablation procedures

In a Cochrane review,[32] it was suggested that there is insufficient evidence to recommend the use of pelvic neuroablation in the management of dysmenorrhoea, regardless of cause. Considering how often laparoscopic uterine nerve ablation has been performed in recent years, it is surprising there has been so little in the way of well-designed, randomised, controlled trials. A small, randomised, double-blind, prospective study was published in 1987 by a team from Detroit, USA,[71] which included only 21 women. It compared, in women with primary dysmenorrhoea, LUNA with diagnostic laparoscopy only. Although LUNA showed effectiveness in the short term, this appeared to decline over time. In 1996, Chen et al.[42] confirmed this observation and demonstrated that laparoscopic presacral neurectomy may retain its effectiveness for a longer period of time but, as mentioned above, there are a considerable number of unpleasant side effects.

The Guildford Birthright Trial[20] described above had a major flaw in that all women in the treatment arm had laparoscopic uterine nerve ablation as well as laser vaporisation of all visible endometriotic implants. This inevitably attracted criticism on the basis that there was uncertainty as to which of these procedures contributed to the overall good results. We have recently completed a further randomised, double-blind, prospective trial of 51 patients, in which one group had LUNA plus laser vaporisation of endometriosis, while the control group merely underwent laparoscopic laser vaporisation of endometriosis without any denervation procedure. At six months follow-up, it was found that the LUNA procedure did not confer any additional benefit to the overall good result, which was almost the same as the result of our original randomised, controlled trial.[72] Vercellini *et al.* came to the same conclusion in a randomised, prospective study with 81 patients.[73] It is interesting to speculate on the overall good results obtained with LUNA in our original retrospective study.[74] A possible explanation is that many women with severe dysmenorrhoea do have deep infiltration of the uterosacral ligaments and the large laser crater, measuring about 20 mm in diameter and 5–10 mm in depth, clearly must have removed a lot of this abnormal tissue, which is known to give rise to severe pain. We are increasingly seeing young women with deeply infiltrating endometriosis running laterally from the rectovaginal septum or a nodule posterior to the cervix, which then infiltrates laterally into the uterosacral ligaments and sometimes even into the pelvic sidewall.

Radical excision of the uterosacral ligaments, either with a CO_2 laser or with electrosurgery, is becoming more and more common, and because the tissue removed is similar to a bull's horn, the operation is called the arcus taurinus procedure. Using this technique, Jean Bernard Dubuisson and his team produced dysmenorrhoea relief in 46 of 50 women (92%) and dyspareunia relief in 47 of 51 women (92%).[75] They noted that the revised AFS score[21] bore no correlation with the symptoms and concluded that this scale for disease severity is only of value in women with infertility. The also noticed that the treatment was equally efficacious, whether or not the histology showed endometrial glands and stroma. In almost 50% of cases, these were not present and the pathological finding was that of fibromuscular hyper-plasia. This observation makes nonsense of the criticism that laser vaporisation of uterosacral ligament disease is inferior to *en bloc* dissection since it does not provide an histological specimen. We disagree with this criticism because it is obvious to see the white fibromuscular hyperplasia and the surgeon continues vaporising until normal tissue becomes visible. Using this technique, we get similar results to those of other teams applying electrosurgery, but our technique takes between 40 minutes and an hour, whereas radical excision can take two or three times as long.

Radical surgery: total hysterectomy and bilateral salpingo-oophorectomy

Although most studies of laparoscopic laser surgery show pain relief in about 70% of treated women, there remains the difficult problem of how to manage the failures. In the long-term follow-up of patients enrolled in the Guildford Birthright

Study,[20] referred to above, we found that six women eventually came to hysterectomy, but there was no sign of endometriosis either macroscopically or microscopically, and sadly, hysterectomy did not relieve their pain. It is imperative to rule out other causes of pelvic pain, particularly when second-look laparoscopy does not show any sign of residual disease.

Most of our work has been in the development of conservative surgery due to the fact that the patient population is often a very young one and many of these women have not yet completed their families. Nevertheless, in a number of women, the only realistic solution to the pain and misery inflicted by endometriosis is to perform a pelvic clearance, which includes a total abdominal hysterectomy and bilateral salpingo-oophorectomy with removal of all active deposits of endometriosis. It is illogical to conserve one ovary on the basis of a woman's young age because the oestrogens are the growth stimulus for ectopic endometrial tissue. If any ovarian tissue remains, the disease is likely to recur in as many as 40% of women at five years' follow-up.[76] More important is the fact that, if ovarian tissue is conserved at the time of hysterectomy for endometriosis, 25% of the women will require subsequent laparotomies, often more than once.[77] At the initial surgery, the ovary is often free and mobile but, as the disease process continues, it gets increasingly bound down to the ovarian fossa by dense adhesions. This is a particularly perilous location because the ureter is very close and attempts to remove the ovary are fraught with difficulty and often lead to incomplete removal – the ovarian remnant syndrome – whereby a small nub of ovarian tissue remains and secretes sufficient oestrogen to encourage proliferation of further deposits of endometriosis.

It is crucial to explain to the woman that conservation of the ovary will often result in recurrent disease and that a more logical approach is to remove the ovaries and give immediate hormone replacement, initially as an implant (oestradiol, 50 mg; testosterone, 100 mg) inserted in the abdominal fat at the time of wound closure.[78] Subsequently, hormone replacement can be continued with oestradiol alone in the form of implants, transdermal patches, or oral preparations. The addition of cyclical progesterone is unnecessary; indeed, it may be positively harmful because it could lead to further growth and bleeding from any residual implants.

Ovarian endometriomas – 'chocolate cysts'

There is considerable controversy over the pathogenesis and surgical management of

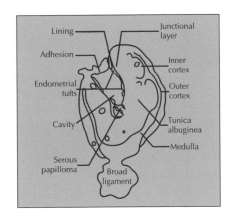

Figure 5.10 *Sagittal section of an endometrioma showing invagination of the cortex due to bleeding from the ovarian fossa. The inside of the 'chocolate cyst' is therefore the outside of the ovarian cortex. (From Hughesdon PE, 1957; with permission.[81])*

ovarian endometriomas, which are also know as 'chocolate cysts'.[79,80] As long ago as 1957, the British pathologist Hughesdon suggested that bleeding from endometriotic implants on the posterior surface of the ovary causes the ovary to adhere to the peritoneum of the ovarian fossa. Furthermore, subsequent bleeding into this space enclosed by adhesions traps the blood, resulting in invagination of the ovarian cortex as the endometrioma enlarges (Figure 5.10).[81]

The majority of ovarian endometriomas appear to fit into this category, since they are densely stuck to the peritoneum of the broad ligament, close to the ureter, and have to be freed by laparoscopic blunt dissection with a strong stainless steel probe, sometimes they have to be divided using laparoscopic scissors. The ovary is gradually levered upwards away from the ovarian fossa, and during this process it invariably ruptures. The haemosiderin-laden fluid is then aspirated and the wound irrigated until the effluent runs clear. In our department, the whole of the inside of the endometrioma is then photo-coagulated with the emerald green KTP/532 laser, which penetrates only a few millimetres, causing only minimal damage to developing follicles under the surface. If a KTP/532 laser is not available, then superficial coagulation can be achieved by using a bicap endocoagulator, which attaches to the suction and irrigation equipment and is relatively simple and safe to use.

An alternative technique is to initially aspirate the endometrioma at the first diagnostic laparoscopy procedure or under ultrasound control and then give the patient GnRH analogues for three months, after which time the shrunken endo-

metrioma will have a relatively avascular capsule that can be vaporised effectively with the CO_2 laser. This particular laser will cause little damage to the developing follicles under the fibrous surface of the capsule, but it does not work in the presence of the haemosiderin-laden fluid of the 'chocolate cyst'.[82,83]

Some laparoscopic surgeons advocate stripping out the ovarian-cyst capsule by traction and counter-traction. In the case of a true endometrioma, this merely results in stripping out the ovarian cortex and leads to profuse bleeding, which requires bipolar coagulation for control and the consequent build-up of heat results in damage to the developing oocytes beneath the surface. It is important to realise that not all 'chocolate cysts' are endometriomas; the 'chocolate' material merely represents haemosiderin and is a reflection of internal bleeding into the cyst. In most of these situations, the ovary is not adherent to the posterior leaf of the broad ligament but is suspended free from the mesovarium and often represents a benign cyst with internal haemorrhage, a haemorrhagic corpus luteal cyst or, occasionally, an endometrioma that has arisen from coelomic metaplasia of invaginated epithelial inclusions.[84–86]

We reported our results on 165 women who presented with large endometriomas, more than 3-cm in diameter.[47] In this study, we used either the CO_2 or the KTP laser and achieved a pain resolution rate of 74% and a pregnancy rate of 45%, but we noticed that there was a higher recurrence rate (30%) in those treated with the CO_2 laser than in those treated with the KTP laser (12.5%).

It is well known that adhesions are more likely to form following laparotomy than laparoscopic surgery.[87–89] Findings from experimental animal studies have been supported by clinical data from a randomised trial, in which adhesions were assessed at second-look laparoscopy following either laparotomy or laparoscopic surgery in the treatment of tubal pregnancy. The results showed much less adhesion formation in the laparoscopy group.

Table 5.1 *Recurrence rates following the laparoscopic management of the endometrioma*

Cyst fenestration and vaporisation

Author	Year	n	Follow-up (months)	Medication	Recurrence rate (%)
Marrs[92]	1991	31	6	Yes	3.2
Fayez[89]	1991	30	2	Yes	33
Donnez[03]	1996	814	2–11 years	Yes	8
Brosens[93]	1996	18	30.5	Nil	0
Sutton[47]	1997	165	6	Nil	12.5–30.0
Hemmings[94]	1998	80	36	Nil	8
Baretta[95]	1998	64	24	Nil	6.2
Saleh[96]	1999	70	18	Nil	21.9

Cyst excision or stripping

Author	Year	n	Follow-up (months)	Medication	Recurrence rate (%)
Bateman[97]	1994	36	12	Nil	11.1
Marana[98]	1994	42	21	Nil	7
Muzzii[99]	1996	21	12	Nil	4.8
Montanino[100]	1996	11	12	Nil	11.1
Beretta[95]	1998	32	24	Nil	6.2
Hemmings[94]	1998	23	36	Nil	12
Saleh[96]	1999	161	18	Nil	6.1
Fayez[89]	1991	66	2	Yes	0–29[a]
Cannis[87]	1992	42	3–6	Yes	7.6[b]
Marana[98]	1994	40	21	Yes	10
Muzzii[99]	1996	20	12	Yes	5
Montanino[100]	1996	25	12	Yes	11.1
Gurgan[88]	1996	19	3	Yes	5.2
Busacca[101]	1999	366	48	Yes	11.7

[a] *all endometriomas < 2 cm in diameter;*
[b] *2 endometriomas (3.8%) < 3 cm in diameter; n = number of women)*

Author	Year	n	Intervention (months)	Pregnancy rate (%)
Daniell[102]	1991	32	Laser ablation and cyst stripping	44
Marrs[92]	1991	23	KTP laser ablation	30.4
Bateman[97]	1994	36	Cyst stripping	42.8
Gurgan[88]	1996	19	Cyst stripping plus GnRH analogue	42.8
Montanino[100]	1996	13	Cyst stripping plus GnRH analogue	45
Donnez[82]	1996	814	CO_2 laser ablation plus GnRH analogue	51
Sutton[47]	1995	24	CO_2 and KTP laser vaporisation	57
Hemmings[94]	1998	84	Cyst stripping versus electrocoagulation	50–60
Beretta[95]	1998	26	Cyst stripping versus electrocoagulation	66.7–23.5
Busacca[101]	1999	366	Cyst stripping	55.4

Table 5.2 *Pregnancy rates following laparoscopic management of the endometrioma*

n = number of infertile women

The cyst recurrence rates following ablative and excisional surgery are shown in Table 5.1, and the pregnancy rates reported in the literature are listed in Table 5.2. The clinical success of each technique in terms of cyst recurrence, pregnancy rates, pain relief and patient satisfaction are only broadly similar. However, this may reflect study design and, in particular, variable follow-up periods and different methods used to document outcome measures.

Follicular reserve

There are concerns about the effect of cyst excision on follicular reserve, due to the probable pathogenesis of endometriomas. It is not unusual to find oocytes in the vicinity of the endometrioma.[83] Furthermore, changes in ovarian artery blood flow have been reported following laparoscopic stripping.[90] A retrospective, controlled study, investigating the follicular response of ovaries after laparoscopic ovarian cystectomy for endometriotic cysts, found

that the follicular response in natural and in clomiphene citrate-stimulated cycles for women older than 35 years was reduced; however, if gonadotrophins were used, the response was comparable.[91] The long-term outcome of this type of surgery on ovarian function is unknown. The loss of follicular reserve may, in theory, precipitate an early menopause.

Evidence based laparoscopic surgery for endometriotic cysts and the Guildford experience.

A logistic regression analysis comparing laparoscopic excision with ablation for endometriotic cysts has been carried out, and compared to the results from our own unit.[103]

Four comparative studies[89,94–96] were identified where cyst recurrence rates were an outcome measure. Cyst recurrence, (%, ±SE) was twice as likely for the ablation treatment (26.6%, ±0.032) than for the excision treatment, (13.2%, ±0.019), ($P < 0.005$, relative risk 1.9). Cyst recurrence following ablative surgery using our technique is comparable (12.6% per cyst and 16.7% per patient)[104] to the pooled rate for excisional surgery. Two comparative studies[94,95] were identified where post procedure pregnancy rates were an outcome measure. Post operative pregnancy rates (%, ±SEM) were not significantly different for the ablation treatment (41.6 %, ±0.138) than for the excision treatment (56.9%, ±0.23). The cumulative pregnancy rate in our series (39.5%)[105] is comparable to the best rates in the literature for either technique. There is only one comparative study to investigate symptom relief,[95] therefore logistic regression analysis is not possible. In our series the "mean temporal changes in pain scores" demonstrated a significant improvement.[106] Three studies[98–100] have compared excisional surgery and peri operative medication with excisional surgery only. The out come measure was cyst recurrence in all three studies. Cyst recurrence rates (%, ±SEM) were not significantly different for group who received medication (10.3 %, ±0.033) than for those that did not (4.0 %, ±0.02). A national survey (UK) was carried out to determine how endometriomas are managed.[107] This demonstrated equal preference for open vs endoscopic surgery. However, 94.7% gynaecologists who perform open surgery carried out ovarian cystectomies, while 50% of minimal access surgeons do not.

REFERENCES

1 Semm K. Tissue puncture and loop ligation – new aids for surgical therapeutic pelviscopy (laparoscopy), endoscopic intra-abdominal surgery. *Endoscopy* 1978; 10: 119–24.

2 Semm K. New methods of pelviscopy (gynecological laparoscopy) for myomectomy, ovariectomy, tubectomy and adnectomy. *Endoscopy* 1979; 11: 85–93.

3 Bruhat M, Mage G, Manhez H. Use of carbon dioxide laser via laparoscopy. In: Kaplan I, editor. *Laser Surgery III. Proceedings of the 3rd Congress for the International Society for Laser Surgery.* Tel Aviv: International Society for Laser Surgery; 1979. p275–82.

4 Daniell JF, Brown DH. Carbon dioxide laser laparoscopy: initial experience in experimental animals and humans. *Obstet Gynecol* 1982; 59: 761–4.

5 Sutton CJG. Initial experience with carbon dioxide laser laparoscopy. *Lasers Med Sci* 1986; 1: 25–31.

6 Donnez J. Carbon dioxide laser laparoscopy in infertile women with endometriosis and women with adnexal adhesions. *Fertil Steril* 1987; 48: 390–4.

7 Luciano AA, Maier D, Koch E, Nillsen J, Whitman F. A comparative study of post-operative adhesions following laser surgery by laparoscopy versus laparotomy in the rabbit model. *Obstet Gynecol* 1989; 74: 220–4.

8 Menzies D, Ellis H. Intra-abdominal adhesions and their prevention by topical tissue plasminogen activator. *J R Soc Med* 1989; 82: 534–5.

9 Macdonald R, Sutton CJG. Adhesions and laser laparoscopic adhesiolysis. In: Sutton CJG, editor. *Lasers in gynaecology.* London: Chapman & Hall, 1992: 95–118.

10 Raftery AT. Effect of peritoneal trauma on peritoneal fibrinolitic activity and intraperitoneal adhesion formation. An experimental study in the rat. *Eur Surg Res* 1981; 13: 397–401.

11 Evers JLH. The pregnancy rate of the no-treatment group in randomised clinical trials of endometriosis therapy. *Fertil Steril* 1989; 52: 906–8.

12 Waller KG, Shaw RW. Gonadatropin-releasing hormone analogues for the treatment of endometriosis: long-term follow-up. *Fertil Steril* 1993; 59: 511–5.

13 Redwine DB. Conservative laparoscopic excision of endometriosis by sharp dissection: life table analysis of re-operation and persistent or recurrent disease. *Fertil Steril* 1991; 56: 628–34.

14 Davis GD. Management of endometriosis and its associated adhesions with the CO2 laser laparoscope. *Obstet Gynecol* 1986; 68: 422–5.

15 Feste JR. Laser laparoscopy: a new modality. *J Reprod Med* 1985; 30: 413–18.

16 Sutton CJG, Hill D. Laser laparoscopy in the treatment of endometriosis. A five-year study. *Br J Obstet Gynaecol* 1990; 97: 181–5.

17 Lomano JM. Nd:YAG laser ablation of early pelvic endometriosis: a report of 61 cases. *Lasers Surg Med* 1987; 7: 56–60.

18 Keye WR, Dixon J. Photocoagulation of endometriosis by the Argon laser through the laparoscope. *Obstet Gynecol* 1983; 62: 383–6.

19 Daniell JF, Miller W, Tosh R. Initial evaluation of the use of the potassium-titanyl-phosphate (KTP/532) laser in gynecologic laparoscopy. *Fertil Steril* 1986; 46: 373–7.

20 Sutton CJG, Ewen SP, Whitelaw N, Haines P. Prospective, randomised, double-blind, controlled trial of laser laparoscopy in the treatment of pelvic pain associated with minimal, mild and moderate endometriosis. *Fertil Steril* 1994; 62: 696–700.

21 The American Fertility Society. Revised American Fertility Society classification of endometriosis: 1985. *Fertil Steril* 1985; 43: 351–2.

22 Sutton CJG, Nair S, Ewen SP, Haines P. A comparison between the CO2 and KTP lasers in the treatment of large ovarian endometriomas. *Gynecol Endosc* 1993; 2: 113–xxx.

23 Revill SI, Robinson JO, Rosen M, Hogg MIJ. The reliability of a linear analogue scale for evaluating pain. *Anaesthesia* 1976; 31: 1191–6.

24 Fedele L, Bianchi S, Bocciolone L, Ni Nola G, Franchi D. Buserilin acetate in the treatment of pelvic pain associated with minimal and mild endometriosis: a controlled study. *Fertil Steril* 1993; 59: 516–21.

25 Sutton CJG, Pooley AS, Ewen SP, Haines P. Follow-up report on randomised controlled trial of laser laparoscopy in the treatment of pelvic pain associated with minimal to moderate endometriosis. *Fertil Steril* 1997; 68: 1070–4.

26 D'Hooghe TM. Natural history of endometriosis in baboons. Is endometriosis an intermittent and/or progressive disease? In: Venturini PL, Evers JLH, editors. *Endometriosis: basic research & clinical practice.* Carnfourth: Parthenon Publishing; 1998. p51–8.

27 Jones KD, Haines P, Sutton C. A long-term follow-up report on a controlled trial of laser laparoscopy for pelvic pain. *J Soc Laparoendosc Surg* 2001; 5: 111–7.

28 Cotte G. Resection of the presacral nerve in the treatment of obstinate dysmenorrhea. *Am J Obstet Gynecol* 1937; 33: 1034–40.

29 Tucker AW. Evaluation of presacral neurectomy in the treatment of dysmenorrhoea. *Am J Obstet Gynecol* 1947; 53: 336–40.

30 Ingersoll F, Meigs JV. Presacral neurectomy for dysmenorrhea. *New Engl J Med* 1948; 238: 357–9.

31 Doyle JB. Paracervical uterine denervation for dysmenorrhoea. *Trans New Eng Obstet Gynecol Soc* 1954; 8:143–6.

32 Johnson N, Wilson M, Farquhar C. Surgical pelvic neuro-ablation for chronic pelvic pain. A systematic review. *Gynecol Endosc* 2000; 9: 351–61.

33 Owman C, Rosenbren E, Sjoberg NO. Adrenergic innovation of the human female reproductive organs: a histochemical and chemical investigation. *Obstet Gynecol* 1967; 30: 763–73.

34 Frankenhauser G. Die Bewegungsnerven der Gebärmutter. *Z Med Nat Wiss* 1864; 1: 35–9.

35 Campbell RM. Anatomy and physiology of sacro-uterine ligaments. *Am J Obstet Gynecol* 1950; 59: 1–5.

36 Latarjet A, Roget P. Le plexus hypogastrique chez la femme. *Gynecol Obstet* 1922; 6: 225–8.

37 Davis GD. Uterine prolapse after laparoscopic uterosacral transection in nulliparous airborne trainees. A report of three cases. *J Reprod Med* 1996; 41: 279–82.

38 Good MC, Copas PR Jr, Doodey MC. Uterine prolapse after laparoscopic uterosacral transection: a case report. *J Reprod Med* 1992; 37: 995–6.

39 Biggerstaff ED. Laparoscopic surgery for pelvic pain. In : Sutton CJG, Diamond M, editors. *Endoscopic surgery for gynaecologists* (2nd edition). London: WB Saunders; 1998. p261–71.

40 Daniell JF, Lalonde CJ. Advanced laparoscopic procedures for pelvic pain and dysmenorrhoea. (Review). *Baillieres Clin Obstet Gynaecol* 1995; 9: 795–808.

41 Nezhat C, Nezhat F. A simplified method of laparoscopic pre-sacral neurectomy for the treatment of central pelvic pain due to endometriosis. *Br J Obstet Gynaecol* 1992; 99: 659–63.

42 Chen FP, Chang SD, Chu KK, Soong YK. Comparison of laparoscopic presacral neurectomy and laparoscopic uterine nerve ablation for primary dysmenorrhea. *J Reprod Med* 1996; 41: 463–6.

43 Candiani GB, Fedele L, Vercellini P, Bianchi S, Di Nola G. Presacral neurectomy for the treatment of pelvic pain associated with end controlled study. *Am J Obstet Gynecol* 1992; 167: 100–3.

44 Marcoux S, Maheux R, Berube S. Laparoscopic surgery in infertile women with minimal or mild endometriosis. Canadian Collaborative Group on endometriosis. *New Engl J Med* 1997; 337: 217–22.

45 Parazzini F. Ablation of lesions or no treatment in minimal–mild endometriosis in infertile women; a randomised trial. Groupo Italiano per lo Studio dell'endometriosi. *Hum Reprod* 1999; 14: 1332–4.

46 Sutton CJG, Ewen SP. Abstract to the International Society of Gynecological Endoscopy Meeting, Washington, DC, 1992: 73.

47 Sutton CJG, Ewen SP, Jacobs SA, Whitelaw NL. Laser laparoscopic surgery in the treatment of ovarian endometriomas. *J Am Assoc Gynecol Laparosc* 1997; 4: 319–23.

48 Olive DL, Stohs GF, Metzger DA et al. Expectant management and hydrotubation in the treatment of endometriosis associated infertility. *Fertil Steril* 1985; 44: 35–9.

49 Lilford RJ, Dalton ME. Effectiveness of treatment for infertility. *Br Med J* 1987; 295: 6591–2.

50 Hull MGR, Glazener CMA, Kelly NJ, Conway DI, Foster PA, Hinton RA, Coulson C et al. Population study of causes, treatment and outcome of infertility. *Br Med J* 1985; 291: 1693–7.

51 Haney AF, Misukonis MA, Weinberg JB. Macrophages and infertility: oviductal macrophages as potential mediators of infertility. *Fertil Steril* 1983; 39: 310–15.

52 Schenken RS, Mallenack LR. Conservative surgery versus expectant management for the infertile patient with mild endometriosis. *Fertil Steril* 1982; 37: 183–5.

53 Daniell JF. Laser laparoscopy for endometriosis. *Colposc Gynecol Laser Surg* 1984; 1: 185–92.

54 Feste JR. Proceedings of the Second World Congress of Gynaecological Endoscopy. Basel: Karger Publications; 1989.

55 Thomas EJ, Cooke ID. Successful treatment of asymptomatic endometriosis: does it benefit infertile women? *Br Med J* 1987; 294: 1117–19.

56 Telima AS, Puolakka J, Ronnberg L, Kauppila A. Placebo controlled comparison of danazol and high dose medroxyprogesterone acetate in the treatment of endometriosis. *Gynecol Endocrinol* 1987; 1: 13–23.

57 Koninckx PR, Martin D. Treatment of deeply infiltrating endometriosis. *Curr Opin Obstet Gynecol* 1994; 6: 231–41.

58 Koninckx PR, Braet P, Kennedy S, Barlow DH. Dioxin pollution and endometriosis in Belgium. *Hum Reprod* 1994; 9: 1001–2.

59 National Centre for Health Statistics. Hysterectomies in the United States 1965–84. Hyattsville M.D. National Centre for Health Statistics, vital and health statistics. Data from the National Health Survey; 1987. Series 13, No 92, DHSS Publ. (PHS) 88–175.

60 World Health Organization. Level of PCBs, PCDDs and PCDFs in breast milk: result of WHO co-ordinated inter-laboratory quality control studies and analytical field studies. *WHO Environmental Health Series.* Geneva: WHO; 1989.

61 Martin DC, Hubert GD, Van der Zwaag R, El Zeky FA. Laparoscopic appearances of peritoneal endometriosis. *Fertil Steril* 1989; 51: 63–7.

62 Holsapple MP, Snyder NK, Wood SC, Morris DL. A review of 2,3,7,8-tetrachlorodibenzo-p-dioxin-induced changes in immunocompetence. *Toxicology* 1991; 69: 219–55.

63 Neubert R, Jacob-Muller U, Stahlmann R, Helge H, Neubert D. Polyhalogenated dibenzo-p-dioxins and dibenzofurans and the immune system. 2. *In vitro* effects of 2,3,7,8-tetrachlorodibenzo-p-dioxin (TCDD) on lymphocytes of venous blood from man and non-human primate (Callithrix jacchus). *Arch Toxicol* 1991; 65: 213–19.

64 Rier SE, Martin DC, Bowman RE, Dmowsky WP, Becker JL. Endometriosis in Rhesus monkeys (Macaca mulatta) following chronic exposure to 2,3,7,8-tetrachlorodibenzo-p-dioxin. *Fundam Appl Toxicol* 1993; 21: 433–41.

65 Reich H, McGlynn F, Salvat J. Laparoscopic treatment of cul-de-sac obliteration secondary to retrocervical deep fibrotic endometriosis. *J Reprod Med* 1991; 3: 516–22.

66 Martin DC. Laparoscopic treatment of advanced endometriosis. In: Sutton CJG, Diamond M, editors. *Endoscopic surgery for gynaecologists.* London: WB Saunders; 1993. p229–37.

67 Martin DC. Laparoscopic and vaginal colpotomy for the excision of infiltrating cul-de-sac endometriosis. *J Reprod Med* 1988; 33: 806–8.

68 Nezhat C, Nezhat F, Pennington E. Laparoscopic treatment of infiltrative rectosigmoid colon and rectovaginal septum endometriosis by the technique of video laparoscopy and the CO2 laser. *Br J Obstet Gynaecol* 1992; 99: 664–7.

69 Redwine DB. Non-laser resection of endometriosis. In: Sutton CJG, Diamond M editors. *Endoscopic surgery for Gynaecologists.* London: WB Saunders; 1993. p220–8.

70 Redwine DB, Sharpe DR. Laparoscopic segmental resection of the sigmoid colon for endometriosis. *J Laparoendosc Surg* 1991; 1: 217–22.

71 Lichten EM, Bombard J. Surgical treatment of primary dysmenorrhoea with laparoscopic uterine nerve ablation. *J Reprod Med* 1987; 32: 37–41.

72 Sutton CJG, Dover RW, Pooley A, Jones K, Haines P. Prospective, randomised, double-blind controlled trial of laparoscopic laser uterine nerve ablation in the treatment of pelvic pain associated with endometriosis. *Gynecol Endosc* 2001 (in press).

73 Vercellini P, Aimi G, Busacca M, Uglietti A, Viganali M, Crossignani PG. Laparoscopic uterosacral ligament resection for dysmenorrhoea associated with endometriosis: results of a randomised controlled trial. (Abstract) *Fertil Steril* 1997; 68 (Suppl 1): 3.

74 Sutton CJG. Laser uterine nerve ablation. In: Donnez J, Nisolle M, editors. *An atlas of laser operative laparoscopy and hysteroscopy.* Louvan: Naucrwclaerts Publishing; 1994. p47–52.

75 Chapron C, Dubuisson JB, Tardif D, Fritel X, Lacroix S, Kinkel K. Retroperitoneal endometriosis and plevic pain: results of the laparoscopic uterosacral ligament resection according to the r-AFS classification and histopathologic results. *J Gynaecol Surg* 1998; 14: 51–8

76 Wheeler JH, Malinak R. Recurrent endometriosis: incidents, management and prognosis. *Am J Obstet Gynecol* 1983; 146: 247–53.

77 Henderson AF, Studd JWW, Watson N. The retrospective study of oestrogen replacement therapy following hysterectomy for the treatment of endometriosis. In: Shaw RW, editor. *Advances in reproductive endocrinology.* Volume 1. Endometriosis. Carnforth: Parthenon Publishers, 1989: 131–40.

78 Sutton CJG. Laparoscopic hysterectomy. *Curr Obstet Gynecol* 1992; 2: 225–8.

79 Jones KD, Sutton CJG. Laparoscopic management of ovarian endometriomas: a critical review of current practice. *Curr Opin Obstet Gynecol* 2000; 12: 309–15.

80 Jones KD, Sutton CJG. Endometriotic ovarian cysts: the case for ablative laparoscopic surgery. *Gynecol Endoscopy* 2001; 10: 281–7.

81 Hughesdon PE. The structure of endometrial cysts of the ovary. *J Obstet Gynecol Brit Emp* 1957; 44: 481–7.

82 Donnez J, Nisolle M, Gillerot S, Anaf V, Clerckx-Braun F, Casanas-Roux F. Ovarian endometrial cysts: the role of gonadotropin-releasing hormone agonist and/or drainage. *Fertil Steril* 1994; 62: 63–6.

83 Donnez J, Nisolle M, Gillet N, Smets M, Bassil S, Casanas-Roux F. Large ovarian endometriomas. *Hum Reprod* 1996; 11: 641–6.

84 Jain S, Dalton ME. Chocolate cysts from ovarian follicles. *Fertil Steril* 1999; 72: 852–6.

85 Nezhat F, Nezhat C, Allan CJ, Metzger DA, Sears DL. Clinical and histologic classification of endometriomas. Implications for a mechanism of pathogenesis. *J Reprod Med* 1992; 37: 771–6.

86 Martin DC, Berry JD. Histology of chocolate cysts. *J Gynecol Surg* 1990; 6: 43–XX.

87 Canis M, Mage G, Wattiez A, Chapron C, Pouly JL, Bassil S. Second-look laparoscopy after laparoscopic cystectomy of large ovarian endometriomas. *Fertil Steril* 1992; 58: 617–19.

88 Gurgan T, Urman B, Yarali H. Adhesion formation and re-formation after laparoscopic removal of ovarian endometriomas. *J Am Assoc Gynecol Laparosc* 1996; 3: 389–92.

89 Fayez JA, Vogel MF. Comparison of different treatment methods of endometriomas by laparoscopy. *Obstet Gynecol* 1991; 78: 660–5.

90 La Torre R, Montanino-Oliva M, Marchiani E, Bonifante M, Montanino G, Cosmi EV. Ovarian blood flow before and after conservative laparoscopic treatment for endometrioma. *Clin Exp Obstet Gynecol* 1998; 25: 12–14.

91 Loh FH, Tan AT, Kumar J, Ng SC. Ovarian response after laparoscopic ovarian cystectomy for endometriotic cysts in 132 monitored cycles. *Fertil Steril* 1999; 72: 316–21.

92 Marrs RP. The use of potassium-titanyl-phosphate laser for laparoscopic removal of ovarian endometrioma. *Am J Obstet Gynecol* 1991; 164: 1622–8.

93 Brosens IA, Van Ballaer P, Puttemans P, Deprest J. Reconstruction of the ovary containing large endometriomas by an extraovarian endosurgical technique. *Fertil Steril* 1996; 66: 517–21.

94 Hemmings R, Bissonnette F, Bouzayen R. Result of laparoscopic treatments of ovarian endometriomas: laparoscopic ovarian fenestration and coagulation. *Fertil Steril* 1998; 70: 527–9.

95 Beretta P, Franchi M, Ghezzi F, Busacca M, Zupi E, Bolis P. Randomised clinical trial of two laparoscopic treatments of endometriomas: cystectomy versus drainage and coagulation. *Fertil Steril* 1998; 70: 1176–80.

96 Saleh A, Tulandi T. Reoperation after laparoscopic treatment of endometriomas by excision and fenestration. *Fertil Steril* 1999; 72: 322–4.

97 Bateman BG, Kolp LA, Mills S. Endoscopic versus laparotomy management of endometriomas. *Fertil Steril* 1994; 62: 690–5.

98 Marana R, Costantini W, Muzzii L, Uglietti A, Caruana P, Arnold M. Laparoscopic excision of ovarian endometriomas: does post-operative medical treatment prevent recurrence? *J Am Assoc Gynecol Laparosc* 1994; 1(4, Part 2): S20.

99 Muzzii L, Marana R, Caruana P, Mancuso S. The impact of preoperative gonadotropin-releasing hormone agonist treatment on laparoscopic excision of ovarian endometriotic cysts. *Fertil Steril* 1996; 65: 1235–7.

100 Montanino G, Porpora MG, Montanino B, Oliva M, Gulemi L, Boninfante M, *et al.* Laparoscopic treatment of ovarian endometrioma. One year follow-up. *Clin Exp Obstet Gynecol* 1996; 23: 70–2.

101 Busacca M, Marana R, Caruana P, Candiani M, Muzzii L, Calia C, *et al.* Recurrence of ovarian endometrioma after laparoscopic excision. *Am J Obstet Gynecol* 1999; 180: 519–23.

102 Daniell JF, Kurtz BR, Gurley LD. Laser laparoscopic management of large endometriomas. *Fertil Steril* 1991; 55: 692–5.

103 Jones KD, Wright JT. Ablative or laparoscopic surgery for endometriotic cysts: resolving the issue. Journal of the American Association of Gynecologic Laparoscopists (In press).

104 Jones KD, Sutton CJG. Recurrence of chocolate cysts after laparoscopic ablation. *Journal of the American Association of Gynecologic Laparoscopists* 2002; 9: 27–32.

105 Jones KD, Sutton CJG. Pregnancy rates following ablative laparoscopic surgery for endometriomas. *Hum Reprod* 2002: 17: 782–785.

106 Jones KD, Sutton CJG. Patient satisfaction and changes in pain scores, after ablative laparoscopic surgery for stage III–IV endometriosis and endometriotic cysts. *Fertil Steril* 2003;: 79: 1086–1090.

107 Jones KD, Fan A, Sutton CJG. The ovarian endometrioma: why is it so poorly managed ? A survey of gynaecological practice in the UK. *Hum Reprod* 2002; 17: 845–849

CONCLUSION

endometriosis until such a time, that science elucidates the cause of the condition, allowing a more logical approach aimed at the prevention of this strange and difficult disease.

The last decade of the 20th century witnessed a revolution in technological progress and surgical skill in the field of minimal-access operative laparoscopy in gynaecology. Most of this effort has been directed towards conservative surgery to improve fertility, but recently, there has been a discernible trend to perform curative radical surgery by laparoscopy. Laparoscopic surgery can be employed for minimal peritoneal endometriosis as well as the most severe stages of the disease. Dense, fibrotic, infiltrative disease of the rectovaginal septum or pelvic sidewall, with retroperitoneal dissection of the ureter can be performed. Laparoscopic surgery is even used to perform segmental resection of the colon involved with endometriosis. Such procedures take a large amount of operating time, and require a skilled and dedicated team to ensure a successful outcome, but the benefits for the patients are enormous. The advantage lies not only in the reduction of postoperative discomfort and the rapid return to normal life, but also because the endoscopic approach is associated with less morbidity, infection, and adhesion formation, which often thwarts the best intentions of the traditional laparotomists.

During the first decade of this century, minimal access endoscopic surgery is likely to continue to expand and develop. It will become the primary treatment for

ENDOMETRIOSIS